Intervolution

NO LIMITS

NO LIMITS

Edited by Costica Bradatan

The most important questions in life haunt us with a sense of boundlessness: there is no one right way to think about them or an exclusive place to look for answers. Philosophers and prophets, poets and scholars, scientists and artists—all are right in their quest for clarity and meaning. We care about these issues not simply in themselves but for ourselves—for us. To make sense of them is to understand who we are better. No Limits brings together creative thinkers who delight in the pleasure of intellectual hunting, wherever the hunt may take them and whatever critical boundaries they have to trample as they go. And in so doing they prove that such searching is not just rewarding but also transformative. There are no limits to knowledge and self-knowledge—just as there are none to self-fashioning.

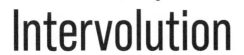

Intervolution

Mark C. Taylor

SMART BODIES
SMART THINGS

Columbia University Press
New York

Columbia University Press
Publishers Since 1893
New York   Chichester, West Sussex
cup.columbia.edu

Library of Congress Cataloging-in-Publication Data
Names: Taylor, Mark C., 1945– author.
Title: Intervolution : smart bodies smart things / Mark C. Taylor.
Description: New York : Columbia University Press, [2020] |
    Series: No limits | Includes bibliographical references and index.
Identifiers: LCCN 2020017703 (print) | LCCN 2020017704 (ebook) |
    ISBN 9780231198202 (hardback) | ISBN 9780231198219
    (trade paperback) | ISBN 9780231552530 (ebook)
Subjects: LCSH: Medical innovations. | Prosthesis. | Human body
    and technology. | Biomedical engineering. | Technology—Social
    aspects.
Classification: LCC RA418.5.M4 T37 2020 (print) | LCC RA418.5.M4
    (ebook) | DDC 610.28/4—dc23
LC record available at https://lccn.loc.gov/2020017703
LC ebook record available at https://lccn.loc.gov/2020017704

Cover design: Lisa Hamm

For
Robin Goland
and her colleagues at the Naomi Berrie Diabetes Center

We have to think of the body plugged into a new technological terrain.

—STELARC

Contents

Preface

Agricultural Revolution. Industrial Revolution. Information Revolution. Internet Revolution. When revolution becomes the normal condition, emergent developments no longer seem revolutionary. Nevertheless, as disruptive technologies appear at an accelerating rate and global networks continue to expand and become more invasive, the world seems to be rushing toward some kind of inflection point. This turn of events provokes both utopian and dystopian visions of the future. For some of Silicon Valley's true believers, new digital and networking technologies are converging with innovations in neuroscience, nanotechnology, and genetic engineering to usher in what has been dubbed "the Singularity," which promises to launch human beings into a new stage of evolution where all ills will be cured and even death will be overcome. Entrepreneurs and investors with more worldly concerns are convinced that the same technologies create the prospect of expanding markets that will generate vast wealth. Many thoughtful critics, however, interpret these developments differently. The optimism of the early days of personal computers and the Internet has given way to anxiety about a panoptical world in which privacy vanishes as personal images and data are bought and used for pernicious economic and political purposes. Technologies that had been promoted as vastly increasing freedom of choice for individuals now threaten the very foundations of democratic societies. As the reach of an invisible network state grows, more and more citizens and politicians are calling for the regulation and even the dismantling of the high-tech companies in which so much hope has recently been invested. Right or left. Red or Blue. Technophilic or technophobic. Utopian or dystopian. As always, both extremes are misleading.

While there is no doubt that digital technologies are changing our minds and bodies in many unpredictable ways, the Promethean dreams of technological gurus like Ray Kurzweil, Jeff Bezos, Elon Musk, and their epigones are, unbeknownst to them, the latest version of Nietzsche's will to power and Heidegger's will to mastery. While a few may thrive, many more struggle and even suffer. When the will to control is out of control, natural processes and disempowered human beings become standing reserves exploited by those who hold the digital advantage. The dreams of some people are the nightmares of others. Technologies that were supposed to unite different people around the world and increase communication and cooperation have turned out to be so divisive they are creating disagreements and conflicts between and among groups that no longer even try to understand each other. Social media, paradoxically, are antisocial. Furthermore, the combination of high-speed computers, networked mobile devices, proliferating cameras and sensors, and Big Data has created a condition of asymmetrical transparency that has led to a surveillance state designed to support surveillance economies. Whereas, in industrial capitalism, those who owned the means of production had the power, in surveillance capitalism, communism, and socialism, those who own the networks and control the data have the power. As the abuses of digital technologies spread, there are louder and louder calls for regulation and reform. A growing number of informed and informative books and articles sound the alarm about current and projected developments. While in no way minimizing the importance of these works, I undertake a different task in this book.

Without a doubt, there is an urgent need for thoughtful assessment and oversight of the technologies that are shaping our future. Effective policies must be developed by people who understand not only the dangers but also the potential for these technologies to improve life and alleviate human suffering. Nowhere are these possibilities greater today than in the area of medical research and development. In the following pages, I will consider some of the ways in which the same image-processing and voice recognition technologies, as well as tracking devices that are being used for political, economic, and even criminal surveillance, and apps that are being used for real and fake targeted political ads and customized marketing are also being used to monitor patients and deliver precision medical care. Networked medical devices monitored by vigilant algorithms are allowing patients to live longer without the debilitating complications that so many terrible diseases often bring. Technology is never neutral—it can always be used for good and for ill. It would be a serious mistake to allow the abuse of advanced information and networking technologies to disrupt medical research and prevent the deployment of digital devices that are already saving lives.

Finally, a word about the title of this book—*Intervolution*. According to the *Oxford English Dictionary*, *intervolve* was first used by John Milton in 1667: "Mazes intricate, Eccentric, intervolv'd, yet regular, Then most, when most irregular they seem." In 1850, Nathaniel Hawthorne used *intervolution* in *The Scarlet Letter*: "Making one little pause, with all its wreathed intervolutions in open sight." *Intervolve* derives from *inter + volvere*, to roll, wind, and means to wind or coil together. In contrast to *evolve*, which means to unfold or rollout (*e*, *ex* + *volvere*), and *coevolve*, which means to evolve jointly or in parallel (*co*, joint, together + *volvere*), *intervolve* means to intertwine. Intervolution involves a developmental process in which seemingly distinct entities are braided together in such a way that each becomes itself in and through the other and neither can be itself apart from the other. Though the word is old, it accurately captures something new about the interplay of smart bodies and smart things in the proliferating webs and networks that constitute our world. Friedrich Nietzsche's words in *Thus Spoke Zarathustra* have never been truer: "All things are entwined, enmeshed, enamored."

Acknowledgments

Researching and writing this book has taken me into new territories and would not have been possible without the generous assistance and support of many people. I would like to express my deep appreciation to Margaret Weyers, Chip Lovett, Bill Lenhart, and Betty Zimmerberg, Williams College; Kevin McCurry, Ittai Dayan, and Mark Michalski, Partners HealthCare; Herbert Allen, Rob Lowe, and John Koski, Allen & Co.; Clark Otley, Mayo Clinic; Gordon and Susan Weir, Joslin Clinic; Rosalind Picard and Ethan Zuckerman, MIT Media Lab; Jack Miles, University of California, Irvine; George Rupp and Wayne Proudfoot, Columbia University; Esa Saarinen, Helsinki; Robin Goland, Remi Creusot, Utpal Pajvani, Rudolph Leibel, Dieter Egli, Cara Lampron, Courtney Melrose, and Megan Sykes, Naomi Berrie Diabetes Center, Wendy Lochner and Costica Bradatan, Susan Pensak, Lisa Hamm, and Lowell Frye of Columbia University Press; and, as always, Dinny Stearns Taylor.

Intervolution

1

Our Bodies Our Selves

I f you can understand the "artificial" pancreas I wear on my belt, you can understand the world now emerging in our midst.

It all begins with disease. Not any disease, but chronic disease, terminal disease. Disease reveals the self you never knew you were and shatters the familiar everyday world by stealing time you once thought was yours. Unexpected words single you out and leave you alone, isolated even from those with whom you are closest. "You are sick, and there is no cure for the disease you suffer. With commitment and discipline it can be managed, and fatal complications can be deferred. At least for a while." In an instant time—lifetime—changes. You withdraw into yourself and look back to the past for an explanation that never satisfies. Why did this happen? Why did it happen now? Could I have done anything to avoid it? More exercise, less meat and sugar? Should I feel shame, guilt, self-pity? What should I say to others? Should I reveal or conceal "my" disease? Will others see me differently? What will they say about me behind my back? Was disease always there, even before I was here, silently lurking in the body of my father or mother, in the bodies of their parents and grandparents? Will I pass on this disease to my children and grandchildren, or will it skip them only to reappear in generations neither I nor they will ever know? Is biology destiny? Was my future always already programmed in a code I did not write?

As the past overwhelms the future, the present is transformed. I gradually realize that I am not and never have been who I thought I was. More precisely, I have always been and always will be both myself and the other of myself. The problem is not, as religious believers and philosophers have long insisted, mind vs. body, but, rather, body vs. body. The duplicity of consciousness and self-consciousness reflects a divided body. This fault cannot be mended, this gap cannot be closed, this tear cannot be wiped away. There is no cure—my condition cannot be changed; it is permanent and must be accepted, and the attempt to deny it only makes it worse. The diagnosis of the other must become my own. My doctor's words "You are" must be repeated as "I am." "I am sick, and there is no cure for the disease I suffer. With commitment and discipline, I can manage my condition and defer fatal complications. At least for a while." Acceptance is not resignation; to the contrary, acceptance makes it possible to utter Samuel Beckett's words again and again, "I can't go on, I'll go on."[1]

Chronic disease is relentless—it never takes a holiday. Year after year, month after month, week after week, day by day, hour by hour, minute by minute, illness must be managed. What makes the disease so pernicious is that its symptoms are not always visible, and, thus, others cannot understand what you are dealing with unless you decide to reveal your secret to them. How can you tell them that the thread of your life has unraveled and you have discovered that you are not who you thought you were? How can you explain to them that you can no longer do what you once did? While they are eating, drinking, playing, dancing, you are always silently counting, calculating, adjusting. The unavoidable repetition compulsion, which management requires, makes it difficult to connect the dots of one's life to form a coherent narrative that extends from the past through the present to the future or, conversely, from the future through the present to the past. Life and death become as much quantitative as qualitative.

For Pythagoras, numbers were the substance of things seen and unseen—pure forms that can be mathematically defined transcend space and time yet nonetheless constitute the program on which the world runs. For those who know the code, nothing remains mysterious. If analysis is careful and calculation is precise, numbers explain everything. Though this ancient faith still has many followers, I have always been skeptical. Do numbers tell the whole story? What if things are not so precise? Is life actually quantifiable? Is it numbers all the way down and all the way in? Can everything be measured? Everyone calculated? Can every code be broken? Every program debugged? Questions proliferate endlessly until disease—chronic disease—befalls you, and then everything changes. Numbers that yesterday were meaningless today are a matter of life and death. Numbers, countless numbers: 120/80 (blood pressure), 80–120 (glucose), below 7 (glycohemoglobin), below

200 milligrams per deciliter (HDL cholesterol), below 100 (LDL cholesterol), 8,000–12,000 (white blood cell count), 12 million (red blood cell count), below 3.5 grams per deciliter (albumin), 135–144 milliequivalent per liter (sodium), .06–1.2 milligrams for every deciliter of blood (creatinine). Normalcy you discover is a very narrow bandwidth. Too much or too little, too high or too low, and the system shuts down. At the tipping point, the rising and falling line on the graph charting vital statistics flatlines. Whether waking or sleeping, adjustments constantly must be made. Far from a dumb machine or mindless meat, the body is incomprehensibly smart. It is an astonishing information-processing network of networks that continuously makes innumerable calculations even the most accomplished scientists do not fully understand. When a circuit breaks or a part malfunctions, the patches applied, implants inserted, and prostheses attached struggle to mimic processes that are only imperfectly understood. No matter how hard you try, life always remains out of balance. Struggling with chronic disease becomes frustrating and wears you down; many days it all becomes too much, and you just want to give up.

O O O

On April 4, 1967, Martin Heidegger delivered a lecture with the daunting title "The Provenance of Art and the Destination of Thought" in Athens. It quickly becomes apparent that he is more concerned with technology than with art, though he sees the two as inseparable. Writing during the Cold War with the overshadowing threat of atomic annihilation and at the dawn of the Information Revolution, which

brought the promise and danger of the new era in biotechnology ushered in by James Watson and Francis Crick's
cracking of the genetic code in 1953, Heidegger argues that
modern science and technology bring to full expression the
will to power inherent in the Western philosophical tradition ever since its beginning in ancient Greece. In retrospect, his analysis proves to be astonishingly prescient.
What is most surprising about Heidegger's argument is his
early recognition of the far-reaching implications of cybernetics and information-processing machines. "The fundamental characteristic of the cybernetic blueprint of the
world," he argues, "is the feedback control system, within
which the inductive feedback cycle takes place. The widest
feedback control circle comprises the interactions between
human being and the world." The distinguishing feature of
the techno-social system emerging in the 1950s and 1960s
was the tendency to quantify human behavior in a way that
made it calculable and thus subject to human manipulation and control. It is worth quoting Heidegger's argument
at length because he effectively frames the issues and poses
many of the questions I will consider in the following
pages.

> The cybernetic blueprint of the world presupposes that
> steering or regulating is the most fundamental character-
> istic of all calculable world-events. The regulation of one
> event by another is mediated by the transmission of a mes-
> sage, that is, by information. To the extent that the regu-
> lated event transmits messages to the one that regulated
> it and so informs it, the regulation has the character of a
> positive feedback-loop of information.

This bidirectional movement of the regulation of events in their interdependence is thus accomplished in a circular movement. That is why the fundamental characteristic of the world, in this cybernetic blueprint, is this feedback control system. The capacity for self-regulation, the automation of a system of motion, depends on such a system. The world as represented in cybernetic terms abolishes the difference between automatic machines and living beings. It is neutralized in this indiscriminate processing of information. The cybernetic blueprint of the world ... makes possible a completely homogeneous— and in this sense universal—calculability, that is, the absolute controllability of both the animate and the inanimate world. Humanity also has its place assigned to it within this uniformity of the cybernetic world. . . . Within the purview of cybernetic representation, the place of humankind lies in the widest circuit of the feedback control system. According to the modern representation of man, he is in fact the subject who refers himself to the world as the domain of objects in that he works on them. The ensuing transformation of the world is fed back onto the human being. The subject-object relation, in its cybernetic understanding, consists of the interaction of information, the inductive feedback within the widest circuit of the feedback control system, which can be described by the designation of "man and world."[2]

In this cybernetic feedback loop, human beings create technologies, which, in turn, recreate human beings.

Through this two-way process, a subtle but crucial reversal occurs—the very effort to attain mastery and control by subjecting all natural and worldly processes to human ends turns individuals into prostheses of the machines they create. As Kierkegaard was the first to realize, this process starts with industrialism's mass production and mass media, and, as Heidegger argues, it is extended by cybernetics and later by digital media. Modern technology results in a condition Heidegger labels "everydayness" (*Allta a umlaut glichkeit*). "Everydayness," he explains,

> manifestly stands for that way of existing in which Dasein [i.e., human being] maintains itself "every day." And yet this "every day" does not signify the sum of those "days" which have been allotted to Dasein in its "lifetime." Though this "every day" is not to be understood calendrically, there is still an overtone of some temporal character in the signification of the "everyday." . . . "Everydayness" means the "how" in accordance with which Dasein "lives unto the day." . . . To this "how" there belongs further the comfortableness of the accustomed, even if it forces one to do something burdensome and "repugnant." That which will come tomorrow (and this is what everyday concern keeps awaiting) is "eternally yesterday's." In everydayness everything is one and the same, but whatever the day may bring is taken as diversification.[3]

When "the comfortableness of the accustomed" becomes a person's primary preoccupation, the self is scattered and absorbed in others. Interiority disappears as the public invades the private. No longer thoughtful and responsible subjects, people engage in "idle talk" and mindless chatter in which they do not think for themselves but become vehicles for the noise of mass media. Unique individuality disappears in an anonymous "They" as masses unknowingly avoid anxiety and flee the awareness of death by finding reassurance in everyday routine. What appear to be responsible decisions are really actions programmed by others. Rather than autonomous actors, shoppers on Amazon's website are automatons run by hidden machinations to which they remain blind.

The overriding purpose of Heidegger's entire philosophy is to awaken people from their self-forgetfulness and alert them to their singularity. To explain how self-awareness is cultivated, he offers the unlikely example of a dedicated craftsman whose familiarity with his tools makes them an extension of his body. Like the gifted athlete who is in the zone, the skilled craftsman works unselfconsciously. The absence of deliberation and calculation lends his movements ease, spontaneity, and grace. Past and future disappear in the present moment, which becomes all absorbing—until the tool breaks or is missing. When the spell is broken, the craftsman becomes aware of the tool as a separate object and of himself as an independent agent. Disease—especially serious disease—is the functional equivalent of the tool breaking. In everyday life, the body performs so smoothly that most of the time we remain unaware of it until disease disrupts its rhythms. Chronic and terminal diseases shatter the everyday world and disrupt routines that now appear to have been strategies designed to avoid the prospect of disease and the inevitability of demise. The present is no longer all-consuming because awareness is always divided between a past that has become questionable and a future that remains uncertain.

For Heidegger, the recognition of individuality is most acute in the awareness of death. The death of others makes one aware of one's own impending death and disrupts everything that once had seemed secure. No one can die in my place, and in confronting my mortality I realize that I must accept responsibility for the individual person I have become. In this way, the acknowledgment of death transforms one's relation to time. No longer lost in the present, the self remains suspended between a recollected past that is always receding and an anticipated future that is forever approaching.

The self one discovers when shaken by disease is not precisely the one Heidegger described five decades ago. When you are ill—chronically ill—self-forgetfulness is a luxury you cannot afford. Heidegger was right when he argued that the awareness of death singles you out from others and leaves you standing alone. If you choose life over death, constant vigilance, focused attention, and deliberate self-discipline are required. But Heidegger was wrong when he argued that quantification and calculation are marks of inauthenticity; to the contrary, they are conditions of life itself. The insulin junkie is always counting and calculating—blood glucose, carbs, exercise, doses. Too much or too little insulin results in confusion, disorientation, hallucinations, sometimes coma, and even death. Heidegger was also right about the importance of cybernetics, but was also wrong to insist that expansion of information and communications technologies necessarily leads to the loss of so-called authentic selfhood. Today even a hut on a hillside in the Black Forest is wired to the entire world. This connectivity need not distract the mind and disturb the body; rather, networking mind and body can open new channels for messages that sustain life. Our Bodies Our Selves. Contrary to expectation, just as the acceptance of death creates new possibilities for living, so disease can be surprisingly liberating—by shaking an individual out of his or her lethargy of everydayness, disease expands awareness by revealing life's limits.

O O O

If I had lived one hundred years ago, I would have been dead for more than three decades. As we will see in detail in the next chapter, diabetes is the result of the pancreas producing too little or none of the insulin necessary to metabolize blood glucose or sugar. While ancient Egyptians and Greeks recognized what eventually was named diabetes, it was centuries before scientists began to understand the disease, and even today there are more questions than answers. Effective treatment had to await the discovery of insulin in 1921. Insulin is a hormone produced by cells in the pancreas that regulates the metabolism of carbohydrates, fats, and glucose from the blood in the liver.[4] In 1869, the German physiologist Paul Langerhans discovered the portion of the pancreas responsible for creating the cells that produce insulin. The first person to suggest that pancreatic cells might be involved in controlling blood sugar was the English physiologist Sir Edward Albert Sharpey-Schafer, who is widely regarded as the founder of endocrinology. The real breakthrough came several decades later when Frederick G. Banting, who was a general practitioner working in Canada, became obsessed with finding a cure for diabetes. Prior to his efforts, diabetes was inevitably fatal. The only treatment for the diseased involved a near-starvation diet that required precisely measuring every gram of carbohydrates consumed. Even for those who faithfully followed this strict regimen, the best that could be hoped for was a brief delay of death. Patients were condemned to a slow death as their energy ebbed and their bodies wasted away. Arataeus's description of diabetics in the first century C.E. grimly described their condition as "a melting down of the flesh and limbs into urine."[5] Faculty members at the University of Toronto dismissed Banting as a country bumpkin whose ideas could not compete with the advanced research they were doing. But Banting persisted and eventually persuaded John Macleod to give him laboratory space and a modest stipend with which he bought dogs that he used to conduct his experiments. Eventually, he and his colleague Charles Best were able to remove insulin-producing cells from the pancreas and purify the extract. After trials on dogs, Banting successfully administered insulin to humans, and, for the first time, people with diabetes were no longer necessarily condemned to an early death. In 1923, Banting and Macleod, but not Best, received the Nobel Prize in Physiology or Medicine for the discovery of insulin.

Since Banting's discovery, research has followed two tracks: first, the investigation of the origin, operation, and possible cure for diabetes; second, the search for treatments to mitigate the effects of the disease. I will consider the first line of inquiry in the next chapter; in the following pages I will concentrate on current treatment technologies. A century after its discovery, insulin remains the only drug that can alleviate the symptoms of type 1 diabetes. Today insulin is produced by using recombinant DNA technology in which a human gene is inserted into the genetic material of a common bacterium. In the last hundred years, the therapy for diabetes has remained basically the same, though the method of delivering insulin has changed dramatically. The most significant developments have occurred in the past five to six years. While medical research continues to make steady progress, the most important changes in treatment have been the result of the transfer of new technologies created for very different purposes to medical applications. We are in the midst of major changes in medical research and clinical practice that are part of a much larger technological revolution. When I started treatment for diabetes more than thirty years ago, I had to check my blood six to eight times a day, estimate my carbohydrate consumption, calculate the amount of insulin needed to stabilize my blood glucose, and administer the insulin with an injection. There was no way to ascertain glucose levels between blood tests and there was no way to deliver insulin other than intermittent injections with syringes. In the ten years before I started using an insulin pump, I injected insulin into my body approximately 16,000 times, and in the nearly thirty years before I started using a continuous glucose monitor (CGM), I drew blood to test approximately 65,000 times.

In the absence of a cure, the dream of patients, researchers, and physicians for many years has been an invention that could monitor, regulate, and automate the delivery of insulin: such a device would be, in effect, an artificial pancreas. In 1963, Arnold Kadish created the first insulin pump, which was as big as a heavy backpack.

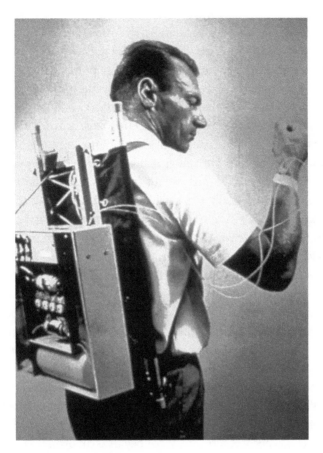

FIGURE 1.1 First insulin pump.

While the size, weight, and cumbersomeness of the machine made it impractical, the experiment provided proof of concept and encouraged further investment and research. The first commercial pump, known as the Big Blue Brick, was introduced in 1978, but its use was restricted because of the difficulty ensuring safe insulin dosage. Throughout the late 1980s and early 1990s, major advances were made in the size, flexibility, and accuracy of pumps. By the time I began using an insulin pump in the late 1990s, it was the size of a phone pager and could be worn on a belt or attached to one's clothing. It was still necessary to test your blood, estimate carbohydrates, and input the grams of carbohydrates consumed. When programmed with the patient's individual insulin sensitivity, the pump would calculate the quantity of insulin needed. The next major advance leading to a viable artificial pancreas was the Food and Drug Administration's approval of the first continuous glucose monitor in 1999. Sensors inserted into the body every seventy-two hours take subcutaneous glucose readings every ten seconds, thereby eliminating the need for finger-prick blood tests. By 2017, this system had been improved so much that sensors could remain in the body for ten days and a transmitter could send data up to twenty feet for display on a handheld receiver or a mobile phone. At the same time that new sensor technology was being developed, pumps were being redesigned to be integrated with continuous glucose monitors. By closing the loop between pump and monitor, the dream of an artificial pancreas has become a reality. What began as an oversize backpack, almost too heavy to carry, became a wearable device considerably smaller than a deck of cards.

The inconspicuous device I wear on my belt is "my" quasi-automatic digital pancreas. It is a small black device that looks like a mobile phone, so no one ever notices it. If you look carefully, however, you can see a translucent plastic tube tucked under my shirt that is connected to another

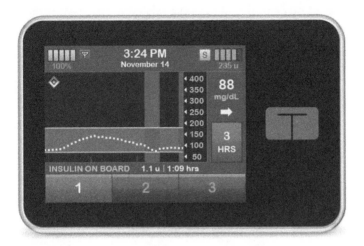

FIGURE 1.2 My insulin pump.

tube inserted in my body. A touch screen displays numbers that indicate the amount of insulin in my body and the length of time it will remain active. There is also a graph plotting dots that register readings from a continuous glucose monitor every five minutes for three, six, twelve, and twenty-four hours. These data are transmitted wirelessly to the pump from the sensor, which I also insert into my body. The horizontal axis of the graph measures blocks of time ranging from three to twenty-four hours, and the vertical axis has numbers from fifty to four hundred, which indicate my glucose level. The dotted line records the increase and decrease in my glucose level. A horizontal red line indicates the lower limit for my glucose, and a horizontal yellow line indicates the upper limit. Using finely tuned algorithms to process the information from the sensor and the pump as well as data accumulated for the past several weeks, the pump calculates whether I need more or less insulin. The only input for this calculation I have to make is the grams of carbohydrates I consume.

There are currently two forms of the artificial pancreas. In the semi-autonomous artificial pancreas, the pump calculates the insulin required and allows the patient to approve and trigger the release of the insulin. The autonomous artificial pancreas is called the closed-loop system because data from the continuous glucose monitor are transmitted directly to the pump, which independently calculates the required dosage and automatically delivers it. Both versions of the pump indicate whether glucose levels are increasing, decreasing, or holding steady and can anticipate problems before they occur. The rate of decrease is calculated in relation to the active insulin in the body, and, when necessary, insulin delivery is suspended. Current systems are especially effective in anticipating low blood glucose levels and interrupting the flow of insulin to prevent complications. In the closed-loop system, the rate of glucose increase is calculated in relation to the amount of insulin in the body and, when necessary, additional insulin is automatically delivered. All these calculations must be precise—too much insulin results in hypoglycemia, which can lead to confusion, hallucinations, loss of consciousness, coma, and death. Too little insulin results in hyperglycemia, which can also result in damage to blood vessels, kidneys, nerves, and organs. Long-term hyperglycemia leads to blindness, neuropathy, kidney failure, heart attack, stroke, and death.

While the autonomous artificial pancreas is a closed-loop system, it is, like the semi-autonomous artificial pancreas, open to machines and networks extending far beyond the individual's body. Both systems are regulated by the algorithmic processing of data collected and not only in the person's pump but also from millions of other patients and stored in computers scattered around the world that are connected in global networks. At regular intervals, I upload my pump's data into the cloud, where my doctor and the manufacturers of the pump and the CGM, as well as anyone else to whom I give my password, can access it. In the near future this data will be transmitted both from and to the pump in real time. Like all cloud-based systems, the data from my digital pancreas can be hacked by anonymous agents lurking anywhere in the world. The danger of hackers transferring funds from my bank account pales in comparison to the danger of hackers programming a fatal dose of insulin or cutting off my insulin supply. Far from a sci-fi fantasy, this is a current danger. In a recent *Wall Street Journal* article entitled "FDA Says Medtronic Insulin Pumps Pose Cybersecurity Risk," Thomas Burton reports, "The Food and Drug Administration warned that certain insulin pumps made by Medtronic PLC have cybersecurity vulnerabilities and could be manipulated by hackers, causing danger to diabetes patients."[6] Though there is much debate about the convenience, reliability, and danger of self-driving cars, trucks, and planes, there is little discussion of the more important creation and proliferation of autonomous digital medical devices that are attached to or implanted in bodies and connected in worldwide webs. If you think going for a ride in a self-driving car requires a leap of faith, try having your life depend on an autonomous pancreas whose algorithms interact with both data in the cloud and information processed by your body's countless interconnected communication networks.

With the move first from mainframe to personal computers and then to handheld mobile devices, there has been a progressive miniaturization, decentralization, and distribution of data-processing machines. The new new thing is the Internet of Things (IoT), which connects scattered devices and enables them to talk to each other. This network links everything from instruments in home security systems and surveillance systems to the Global Position System and servers in high-speed financial networks. In some cases, these connected devices require intentional human interaction, and in other cases the networks operate without human agents. The purpose of the IoT is to collect and analyze data that can be used to control things and through them regulate human behavior.

The same technologies underlying the IoT are also being used to create a newly emerging Internet of Bodies (IoB). Wearable computers like my continuous glucose monitor and insulin pump as well as implantable devices like pacemakers and brain chips are connected through the cloud to remote data-processing centers, where bodily functions and activities are monitored, regulated, and modulated. Bodies distributed in space and time are increasingly interconnected in a worldwide web. The IoT and IoB are inextricably interrelated—each requires the other. When joined together and linked to the Intranet of the Body, they constitute an intervolutionary network in which the form of life following what has been known as humanity is emerging. This global network constitutes the technological unconscious that is the performative infrastructure for bodily and cognitive development in the twenty-first century.

These extraordinary changes are the result of six closely related developments.

1. Ultra-high-speed networked computers
2. Massive quantities of data gathered from the Internet and other sources
3. Expansion of wireless networks
4. Explosive growth of mobile devices
5. Rapid proliferation of low-cost miniaturized sensors
6. Radical changes in artificial intelligence

I will consider each of these developments in the following chapters. In this context, it is important to understand how the interplay of the IoT and the IoB simultaneously extends and modifies technologies and practices that have been operational for more than a century.

It has become commonplace to contrast the so-called Industrial Revolution with the so-called Information Revolution. This is a mistake because the Industrial Revolution was already an Information Revolution, and the Information Revolution is also an Industrial Revolution. Consider, for example, Charlie Chaplin's film *Modern Times* (1936). The film begins with music playing and a full-screen shot of a clock with the second hand moving toward 6:00. After the credits roll, words appear superimposed on the clock. "Modern Times." A story of industry, individual enterprise—humanity crusading in pursuit of happiness." The film captures the travails of workers in post-Depression industrial America. The action begins with a herd of pigs rushing to their slaughter, followed by a herd of men emerging from the subway rushing to a factory, where they assume their assigned positions on the factory floor. While workers desperately scramble to keep up with the assembly line, managers reading newspapers in comfortable offices surrounded by secretaries and calculating machines order their subordinates on the shop floor to keep speeding up production. An elaborate surveillance network of cameras and screens monitors workers even during bathroom breaks. With his bodily movements as automated and mechanized as the production line, Little Tramp rushes to keep up but eventually gets caught in turning gears and is literally devoured.

Chaplin's factory represents the implementation of Frederick Winslow Taylor's *Principles of Scientific Management* (1911), which provided rules and procedures that functioned as algorithms programming workers thereby making them into machines that operate at maximum efficiency. For the industrial system to prosper, mass production required mass consumption, which was promoted through emerging mass media. Modern advertising initially used print media—newspapers, magazines, brochures, pamphlets, and catalogues distributed through the expanding United States Postal Service. With the appearance of radio and television, new advertising agencies devised novel tactics and strategies designed to keep the wheels of production turning. Throughout most of the twentieth century, mass advertising distributed through mass media promoted the mass consumption that mass production required.

During the last two decades of the twentieth century and the first two decades of the twenty-first century, the six innovations I have noted converged to create new forms of production, marketing, and consumption that are more pervasive and invasive. With the ability to gather, store, process, and distribute information about the activities, habits, and patterns of the behavior of individuals in real time, massification gives way to personalization. Mass production and mass advertising are superseded by the mass customization of products and the precision targeting of consumers. The aim of this targeting can be social and political as well as economic. Whatever its purpose, new distributed computational and networking technologies involve, as Heidegger correctly predicted, the quantification, calculation, and modification of human behavior. Charlie Chaplin's managers programming workers on assembly lines have been displaced by closed-loop systems of sensors, embedded in both things and people and run by algorithms on calculating machines trained by machine learning. Information collected by mobile phones and other devices is transmitted to servers where it is processed and personalized by relating it to the previous patterns of an individual's decisions and activities. These data are then retransmitted to the same devices that had sent the original information. Person, device, data center, and computer form a closed loop that is self-generating and self-regulating.

In her timely book *The Age of Surveillance Capitalism: The Fight for a Human Future at the New Frontier of Power*, Shoshana Zuboff, professor emerita at Harvard Business School, writes, "Just as [Henry] Ford tapped into a new mass consumption, Apple was among the first to experience explosive commercial success by tapping into a new society

21

of individuals and their demand for individualized consumption. The inversion implied a larger story of commercial reformation in which the digital era finally offered the tools to shift the focus of consumption from the mass to the individual, liberating and reconfiguring capitalism's operations and assets. It promised something utterly new, urgently necessary, and operationally impossible outside the networked spaces of the digital. . . . In offering consumers respite from an institutional world that was indifferent to their individual needs, it opened the door to the possibility of a new rational capitalism able to reunite supply and demand by connecting us to what we really want in exactly the ways we choose."[7] For many advocates from Silicon Valley to Wall Street, these technologies represent the latest stage in the increasing efficiency of production and consumption that maximizes profits for those who own shares in the means of production and reproduction.

There is, however, a significant price to be paid in terms of privacy and individual autonomy. The intersection of the IoT and the IoB creates what Zuboff aptly labels "Body Rendition." "The rendition of your body begins quite simply with your phone. Even when your city is not 'smart' or owned and operated by Google, market players with an interest in your behavior know how to find your body. . . . Your body is reimagined as a behaving object to be tracked and calculated for indexing and search." Citing a Carnegie Mellon University study of the number of times phone apps accessed location data for a three-week period, Zuboff reports, participants "were flabbergasted by the sheer volume of the onslaught as they each variously learned that their locations were accessed 4,182 times, 5,398 times, 356 times, and so on, over a 14-day period—all for the sake of advertisers, insurers, retailers, marketing firms, mortgage companies and anyone else who pays to play in these behavior markets."[8]

The leader in data processing for targeted advertising, not surprisingly, is Google. As we will see in more detail in chapter 4, everything that is digitized is searchable. Android phones, Gmail, Google Street View, Google Glass, social media, and countless platforms and apps provide data for targeted marketing and behavior modification programs. According to Zuboff, in 2016, 89 percent of the income for Google's parent company, Alphabet, came from targeted advertising. Many of the data for these programs are harvested from the 3.5 billion searchers per day and the 1.2 trillion searches per year. With the exponential expansion of social media, the sources of data are increasing faster than the capacity to process them. Pop-up ads that seemed revolutionary only a few years ago now appear to be a primitive form of much more sophisticated deployments of new technologies. The precision of real-time targeting sometimes is carried to extremes. For example, companies can now adjust automobile insurance rates in real time based upon a person's performance while he or she is driving. If the driver exceeds the speed limit, runs a red light, or fails to stop at a stop sign, the insurance rate goes up, and if he or she complies with the rules of the road, the insurance rate stays the same or even goes down. While continuous rate adjustment might encourage safe driving, the real purpose is undeniably financial—fewer accidents means fewer claims insurance companies must pay, which results in greater profits. In a world that favors innovation and disruption over stability and continuity, there is no end to the effort to monetize data.

What some people regard as an emerging capitalist utopia others see as a looming capitalist or totalitarian dystopia. As computational technologies and AI have become more powerful and miniature cameras and sensors more pervasive, skepticism and criticism of high-speed financial networks, social networks, and Big Data have been increasing. Concern focuses on two primary areas: economic and political. Critics argue that surveillance capitalism effectively combines consumer and finance capitalism by creating high-speed exchange networks where trillions of transactions provide endless data to be mined for economic advantage. To make matters worse, the rise of the Information Revolution has been conterminous with the spread of neoliberal economic principles, which favor unregulated market activity. The cozy relation among Washington, Silicon Valley and Wall Street has created a positive feedback loop accelerating financial returns. This, in turn, has led to the excessive accumulation of capital, which is exacerbating the already large wealth gap. For other critics, the issue is not only the inequitable distribution of wealth and the influence it brings, but also the inequitable distribution of political power. As Marx rightly argued, in industrial capitalism, those who own the means of production hold the power. In today's world, those who own the means of gathering information and processing data hold the power. Asymmetrical transparency is creating a panoptical surveillance state in which ubiquitous cameras, sensors, tracking devices, and facial recognition technology are being used to monitor activity and control people. These developments seem to contradict the original logic of personal computers. As I have noted, the shift from mainframes first to personal computers and then to mobile devices was supposed to create nonhierarchical distributed networks that would facilitate the equitable distribution of wealth and power. However, just as technologies designed to connect us now divide us, so the technologies that were supposed to distribute wealth and power have led to their increasing concentration in the hands of fewer and fewer people.

In 2001, only three years after Google was founded, Larry Page was asked, "What is Google?" "If we did have a category," he responded, "it would be *personal information.* . . . Communications. . . . Sensors are really cheap. . . . Storage is cheap. Cameras are cheap. People will generate enormous amounts of data. . . . Everything you've ever heard or seen or experienced will become searchable. Your whole life will be searchable."[9] When *everything* and *everyone* is searchable, privacy is dead, and, many fear, democracy is doomed. As the unforeseen and unintended consequences of digital technologies become evident, many critics and activists are calling for the strict regulation or even complete dismantling of large technology companies like Google, Microsoft, Apple, Amazon, and Facebook.

Nowhere is the concern about privacy greater than in the area of medical information. Doctors and hospitals have been extremely slow to digitize their records. Everyone is familiar with the frustration of having to fill out the same forms and answer the same questions again and again while doctors, physician's assistants, and nurses slowly write down the information on paper. Further complicating matters, neither different doctors nor different hospitals readily share information. This inefficiency results in enormous losses of valuable time and money. In the past few years, this situation has slowly started to change. Many doctors and hospitals, especially in urban areas, are making the transition from paper to electronic medical records (EMRs), but significant problems still remain. All too often doctors and hospitals use different programs and platforms, and, thus, communication and information transfer are still slow or even impossible. While many of the difficulties are attributable to administrative ineptitude, the reluctance to digitize medical information and standardize data also reflects a justifiable concern with privacy. Many responsible healthcare professionals are worried about the recent entry of large companies like Google, Amazon, and Walmart into the medical business.[10] These ventures assume that business models used in other areas can also disrupt healthcare. Even more valuable than the profits from medical programs is the anticipated value of the accumulated medical data for marketing an expanded range of products. The Internet of Bodies might turn out to be as valuable as the Internet of Things.

Medical information in the hands of companies, employers, colleagues, and even friends and families can have devastating personal, social, and economic consequences. In addition to this, as people become more aware of the ownership, management, sale, and possible misuse of medical information, many are attempting to take control of their data. Companies like PatientSphere, #My31, and Hu -manity.co have created platforms that enable people to limit access to their data and to profit from the use or sale of it.

In February 2019 California governor Gavin Newsom proposed that people should be paid a "data dividend" for the use of their personal information. Senators Mark Werner and Josh Hawley are sponsoring a bill that requires companies to put a price on people's data. Other critics have gone so far as to call for regulating or even dismantling the Big Tech companies responsible for collecting, processing, and selling data.

While these concerns are understandable and, to a certain extent, justifiable, it would be a huge mistake to take precipitous actions that would unduly limit research and technological development by inhibiting the free exchange of medical information. High-speed networked computers, mobile devices, miniature sensors, Big Data, and artificial intelligence are converging to create breakthroughs that offer hope for the treatment and perhaps even the cure of diseases that have plagued human beings for centuries. This work requires the collection, storage, and processing of massive amounts of standardized data. Allowing people to charge for the use of their medical information and excessive regulation would distort the pool of data available to researchers. At the precise moment that research in many areas is approaching the tipping point, overly aggressive policies and regulations threaten to arrest progress. Technology has different costs and benefits in different contexts. The same technologies that enable Amazon to display annoying pop-up ads on your computer screen, or insurance companies to monitor your driving and automatically adjust insurance rates, also make it possible for my insulin pump to continuously monitor my glucose and automatically adjust my insulin dosage in real time. The investigation of the biochemistry of diabetes and emerging strategies for treatment reveal the importance of these technologies for the rapidly expanding Internet of Bodies.

Diabetes is a ticking time bomb in the healthcare systems in many countries today. The growing significance of this disease is not only personal but is also social, political, and economic. In the foreword to the 2017 *IDF Diabetes Atlas,* Shaukat Sadikot, president of the International Diabetes Federation, declares a "current diabetes pandemic." Diabetes, he explains, "is not only a health crisis; it is a global societal catastrophe. Due to its chronic nature, diabetes causes devastating personal suffering and drives families into poverty. Governments worldwide are struggling to meet the cost of diabetes care and the financial burden will continue to expand due to the growing number of people developing diabetes."[11] Currently, 425 million people worldwide, or 8.8 percent of adults between the ages of 20 and 79, have diabetes. This number is predicted to increase to 629 million by 2045. In the past two and a half decades, the incidence of diabetes has almost tripled. The Centers for Disease Control estimates that, by 2050, one in three people in the United States will have type 2 diabetes. Today 4 million people die annually from diabetes and its complications. Alarming as these figures are, they actually underestimate the scope of the problem because 30–80 percent of people with diabetes are undiagnosed.

There are two main types of diabetes: type 1, which is an autoimmune disease and is insulin dependent; type 2, which is not an autoimmune disease and is not insulin dependent. As we will see in the next chapter, both kinds of diabetes involve the malfunctioning of the immune system. In type 1 diabetes, the cells that produce the insulin necessary to metabolize glucose, lactose, fructose, and carbohydrates are destroyed, and survival depends on injecting insulin into the body. In type 2 diabetes, insulin-producing cells are impaired but not destroyed and can produce some but not enough insulin. This condition can be managed by diet, exercise, and oral medication that enhances insulin production.

The occurrence of diabetes is unevenly distributed geographically as well as in terms of age. The countries with the highest incidence of diabetes are China, India, and the United States. The rate of increase is greatest in low- and middle-income countries. Until recently, type 1 was called juvenile diabetes because children were always insulin dependent. Only 7 percent of patients with adult-onset diabetes require insulin. In the past several decades, children have started developing type 2 diabetes.[12] Whether childhood or adult onset, insulin-dependent diabetes occurs almost exclusively in people of European descent. African Americans, Native Americans, and Asians almost never suffer type 1. The rate of type 1 is somewhat higher among Latinos, but remains much lower than among whites, who are by far the most commonly affected ethnicity.

This escalating problem is already creating pressure on healthcare budgets in countries that can least afford it. As of 2017, $720 billion or 12.5 percent of total healthcare costs was spent globally on diabetes. Increasing longevity will further compound the problem. When the age group is expanded to eighteen to ninety-nine years old, the total projected expenditure is estimated to be $958 billion annually. Financial challenges for people with diabetes are

TABLE 1.1 Global Epidemic

Area	Millions of cases 2017	Millions of cases 2045	Percent increase
Western Pacific	159	183	15 percent
South East Asia	82	151	84 percent
Europe	58	67	16 percent
North America and Caribbean	46	62	35 percent
Middle East and North Africa	39	82	110 percent
South and Central America	26	42	62 percent
Africa	16	41	156 percent
World	425	629	48 percent

SOURCE: INTERNATIONAL DIABETES FOUNDATION, 2017

compounded by irresponsible pharmaceutical companies that are cashing in on the pandemic by excessively raising the cost of necessary drugs and medical supplies. There are reports of insulin costing up to $300 per vial. According to Ken Alltucker, "the price of modern versions of a drug that more than 7 million Americans need to live nearly tripled from 2002 to 2013. Type 1 diabetics paid an average of $5,705 for insulin in 2016—nearly double what they paid in 2012."[13] This situation is forcing some patients to ration their insulin and others to travel to countries like

Mexico and Canada where the same bottle of insulin can be purchased for as little as $40 per vial. Many people are being forced to ration their insulin and share syringes. In addition to the cost of insulin, test strips for testing the blood can cost up to $400 a month. The cost of the insulin pump and the continuous glucose monitor system and related supplies is even more extreme:

Insulin pump	$7,250
CGM receiver	$845
Pump cartridges and tubing	$645/three months
Sensors and transmitter	$4,200/three months
Annual cost for pump and CGM supplies	$27,475

31

Given the increasing rate of diabetes, these escalating costs are unsustainable.

Diabetes is not a fashionable disease like AIDS and cancer and thus does not attract athletes and celebrities who purport to show their concern by wearing buttons, ribbons, and pink clothes. This disease involves bodily organs and processes most people prefer to ignore. With dwindling government support, funding for research is increasingly difficult to secure at the precise moment scientists and engineers are on the brink of major breakthroughs. What makes this disease so devastating is that many of its victims are children. While the diagnosis of diabetes is no longer an immediate death sentence, it does condemn its victims to a lifetime of vigilant management, which requires a degree of self-discipline that is difficult to maintain for adults, to say nothing of children and their parents. Diabetes is, nonetheless, a fascinating disease that reveals much about the body and the self as well as social, political, and economic forces at work in the world today.

I have spent my entire professional life trying to understand the human self. Disease, I have suggested, shatters everyday life and forces you to consider yourself and your world anew. Diabetes awoke me from my dogmatic slumber; though I had written many articles and books, it was not until I developed diabetes that I came to appreciate the extraordinary sophistication and complexity of the body. As I have studied the biochemistry of the immune system and autoimmune diseases, I have discovered that scientists and physicians regularly describe diabetes as a "self-other disease." Indeed one popular textbook is entitled *Immunology: The Science of Self-Nonself Discrimination*.[14] Diabetes reveals that the body is smart; more precisely, the body is an intricately calibrated information-processing and communications network of networks that interfaces with the networks of the brain. The body and brain do not form a closed loop; rather, they are connected to networks that extend far beyond their ostensible spatial and temporal boundaries.

The digital pancreas I wear on my belt and the disease it helps me manage transform assumptions about individuals by subverting many of the binary distinctions that have long informed our understanding of ourselves and thereby call into question what it means to be human. Self/Other, Subject/Object, Identity/Difference, Animate/Inanimate, Human/Machine, Natural/Artificial, Body/Mind, Private/Public, Autonomy/Heteronomy. I no longer know what is mine and what is not, and I am no longer sure where "my" body begins and where it ends. Nor am I certain what is living and what is not, or what is inside and what is outside. I do not know who owns "my" pancreas or the data it produces, stores, and transmits. Is all of this "mine"? Or does it belong to the companies that manufacture the continuous glucose monitor and the insulin pump? Do the researchers own the data they mine? Does the insurance company that subsidizes my payments own "my" pancreas and its data? Who owns the intellectual property rights to the algorithms that monitor my glucose and administer my insulin? What happens if these companies go out of business? What happens if the medical supply chain breaks down because the workers go on strike, a hurricane destroys production facilities, a tariff war interrupts exchange, or the plague closes factories? The more interconnected we are, the more fragile we become. Rather than an autonomous individual, I am discovering that I am a shifting node in a network of networks, which forms an Internet of Bodies that is smarter than I ever realized.

2

Intranet of the Body

n *The Sickness Unto Death*, Søren Kierkegaard writes,

As a rule, a person is considered to be healthy when he himself does not say that he is sick, not to mention when he himself says he is well. But the physician has a different view of sickness. Why? Because the physician has a defined and developed concept of what it is to be healthy and ascertains a man's condition accordingly. The physician knows that just as there is merely imaginary sickness there is also merely imaginary health, and in the latter case he first takes measures to disclose the sickness. . . . A physician's task is not only to prescribe remedies, but also, first and foremost, to identify the sickness and, consequently, his first task is to ascertain whether the supposedly sick person is actually sick and whether the supposedly healthy person is actually healthy.[1]

Kierkegaard understood his role to be a physician who diagnoses disease and prescribes medicine for the psychological and spiritual ills people inevitably suffer. His interpretation of health and disease is, like everything else he considers, thoroughly paradoxical. Those who claim to be healthy are actually sick, and those who admit they are sick are on their way to health. Sickness and health are less a matter of either/or than of both/and. In a manner reminiscent of Martin Luther's claim that people are simultaneously justified and sinners, Kierkegaard insists that everyone is both healthy and sick.

Susan Sontag begins her memorable meditation *Illness as Metaphor* by writing, "Illness is the night-side of life, a more onerous citizenship. Everyone who is born holds dual citizenship, in the kingdom of the well and the kingdom of the sick. Although we prefer to use only the good passport, sooner or later each of us is obliged, at least for a spell, to identify ourselves with citizens of that other place."[2] Whenever I go from my Columbia University office at 120th Street and Broadway up to 168th Street, where the Naomi Berrie Diabetes Center is located, I travel from the kingdom of the apparently well to the kingdom of the admittedly ill. The subway bobs below and above ground along the western edge of Harlem. As the stations pass, people get off the train, until most of those remaining are heading to the Columbia University medical complex. Some passengers look sick, most do not. No matter how many times I have made this trip, visiting the clinic is always a sobering experience because it is a stark reminder of the severity of the disease and the dire consequences of not sustaining the rigorous self-discipline the therapeutic regime requires. What is most disturbing, however, is the large number of children, many of whom are African American, who have come for consultation and treatment. They are so young and cannot imagine what lies ahead of them. The lives of the parents, who must help their children cope with the disease, have also been profoundly changed.

Sontag is primarily concerned with the language used to describe disease. "My subject," she writes, "is not physical illness itself but the uses of illness as a figure or metaphor. My point is that illness is *not* a metaphor, and that the most truthful way of regarding illness—and the healthiest way of being ill—is one most purified of, most resistant to, metaphoric thinking. Yet it is hardly possible to take up one's residence in the kingdom of the ill unprejudiced by the lurid metaphors with which it has been landscaped."[3] Sontag's effort is futile—it is impossible to purify thought of images and metaphors. The metaphors we use, which shape the understanding of disease and influence treatment strategies, change with the times and the predominant technologies of an era. While Sontag is most concerned with cancer, tuberculosis, and AIDS, and I am most concerned with diabetes, we share the conviction that the critical awareness of the language we use for illness is important for researchers and physicians as well as patients and the general public.

The metaphorical imagination of disease begins at a very young age. Children have a difficult time understanding disease and need help finding ways to express how their world changes when they become ill. Under the innovative direction of Robin Goland, the Berrie Center has launched the Pancreas Project, which uses art therapy to help children articulate what they cannot say in words. Cara Lampron, who is the leader of the program, meets regularly with individuals and small groups of children, from three years old to adolescents, of diverse racial and ethnic backgrounds. Young patients are encouraged to express their feelings by making drawings. They also sew an artificial pancreas out of felt and tuck notes in it describing how they feel about having the disease. The results of this research are both fascinating and illuminating. The most common response is anger—children feel their pancreas is an enemy that is attacking them. One child declared, "I hate you—you are stupid!" Some children act out this anger by using their felt pancreas as a punching bag. Another child depicted the violence of the disease by drawing his pancreas as an exploding volcano with insulin shooting high into the air. In one case, a child represented diabetes as a war between an angel (a healthy pancreas) and the devil (a sick pancreas). Several children chastised their pancreas for being "lazy" and not wanting to do what it is supposed to do. Many complained that other kids bullied them by calling them names like Robot-Boy, Diabetes-Boy. Though some were initially reluctant to participate in the sessions, most children and parents agree that the program is quite useful. When terms cannot be defined precisely, and distinctions drawn cleanly, language becomes fuzzy and thinking must resort to images and metaphors.

Vestiges of the images and metaphors of children can be detected in the most sophisticated theories and models of scientists. Knowledge is always historically situated and socioculturally conditioned in ways that are often overlooked. From the mechanical clockwork universe of eighteenth-century Deists to the twentieth-century organic universe of believers in the Gaia principle, biological and bodily processes have been interpreted in metaphors that reflect both the changing political situation and new technologies. Though insulin was discovered in 1921, how the immune system and autoimmunity work has only been understood since the end of World War II. In developing their theories, researchers appropriate terms and categories used by the broader scientific community. In the brief history of immunology, six different but interrelated frameworks have oriented research and guided treatment.

Language and semiotics
Cybernetics
Information theory
Military warfare
Alien immigration
Intranet

These different interpretive perspectives are not mutually exclusive; to the contrary, they overlap in such a way that each builds upon the others by updating relevant features in terms of new technologies.

The interpretation of biological and bodily processes in terms of language and semiotics is part of a broader linguistic turn in philosophy and criticism during the first two decades of the twentieth century. Ferdinand de Saussure laid the groundwork for this revolution in his lectures from 1906 to 1911 in Zurich, which were published after his death. Saussure understands language as a system of signs that rests on two basic principles. First, binary opposition defines the structure of every sign. In language, he argues, *identity is difference* because the identity of a particular sign is always constituted by its difference from other signs. Second, every linguistic system consists of two factors: language (*la langue*), which is the underlying structure shared by all speakers, and word or speech (*la parole*), which is the individual event that activates this shared structure. Saussure uses the example of the game of chess to explain how language works.

> But of all comparisons that might be imagined, the most fruitful is the one that might be drawn between the functioning of language and a game of chess. In both instances we are confronted with a system of values and their observable modifications. A game of chess is like an artificial realization of what language offers in a natural form. . . .
>
> First, a state of the chessmen corresponds closely to a state of language. The respective value of the pieces depends on their positions on the chessboard just as each linguistic term derives its value from its opposition to all other terms.
>
> In the second place, the system is always momentary; it varies from one position to the next. It is also true that values depend above all else on an unchangeable convention, the set of rules that exists before a game begins and persists after each move. Rules that are agreed upon once and for all exist in language too; they are the constant principles of semiology.[4]

Just as in chess each piece must be moved according to a specific rule for the match to proceed, so in language particular signifiers must be combined according to a set of formal rules for understanding and communication to occur. In the next chapter we will see that chess not only provides an example of how language works but also serves as the model for the traditional form of artificial intelligence. In this context, it is important to understand how some theoretical biologists have used this account of language to interpret bodily processes in general and the immune system in particular.

In a seminal essay entitled "Signs and Codes in Immunology," published in *The Semiotics of Cellular Communication in the Immune System*," Giorgio Prodi writes, "the semantic dictionary of the immunological code is distributed among a high number of cells, which are in this way different from each other and genetically specific."[5] The translation of the understanding of language as the interplay between structure (language) and event (word/speech) into biological terms is made possible by the introduction of the notion of code, which was invented in the late nineteenth century for telegraphic communication and later adapted to information theory. When communication is understood as the sending and receiving of coded messages, the range of the metaphoric imagination expands. Biological processes now appear to involve active interpretation, which entails both reading and misreading signs. Prodi's analysis again is illuminating.

> If a matter of fact is a sign, the reader for whom such a matter of fact is a sign has a proper code of interpretation, and only on the base of this code the matter of fact is a sign. If a molecular structure is interpreted by the immune

system as an epitope [that is, the part of the antigen or for-eign agent recognized by the immune system] (and is therefore a sign for the system) the question is: how is the code constituted, how does it work to interpret its reality. The mechanism must be based on the general well-established reactions of deciphering (DNA coding, pro-tein synthesis, and so on). Then the question can become the following: how these reactions are combined to pro-duce an "immunological interpretation."[6]

The development of new technologies during and after World War II made this line of argument not only possi-ble but increasingly plausible. It is important to note that much of the early research in computers, cybernetics, and information theory was conducted for military purposes. In England, Alan Turing, who developed a model for a general-purpose computer and is widely considered to be the father of theoretical computer science and artificial intelligence, worked for the Government Code and Cypher School at Bletchley Park. He and his team decoded German cyphers and thereby played a crucial role in the Allied victory in World War II. In the United States, Nor-bert Wiener, who graduated from Tufts University at the age of fourteen and received his Ph.D. with a dissertation on mathematical logic three years later, was the founder of a field he named cybernetics. The word *cybernetics* derives from the Greek *kubernetes* (pilot, governor), which, in turn, stems from *kubernaein* (to steer, guide, govern). The Latin *gubernare* can also be traced to *kubernan*. To govern is to control the action or behavior of someone or some-thing; to guide, direct, administer. But *govern* can also mean to regulate something by determining its speed, pressure, magnitude, or temperature. In his initial research, Wiener was concerned with ballistics, missiles, and weapons systems. He was primarily interested in targeting enemy aircraft and missiles. Wiener named the device he developed for this purpose a *servomechanism,* which operates by negative feedback. By transmitting information and correcting error signals, a servomechanism can control the parameters that determine speed and position of a moving object and adjust the direction and velocity of the missile accordingly. The cruise control device in a car is a more recent example of this kind of regulatory mechanism. When fully developed, cybernetic servomechanisms are self-regulating and can be either autonomous or semi-autonomous. Today's insulin pumps would not have been possible without the invention of these early cybernetic devices.

43

As the range of the application of cybernetics was expanding from mechanical and electronic devices to biological and organic systems, the accurate collection, storage, processing, and transmission of information became necessary. Claude Shannon's important paper, "The Mathematical Theory of Communication," published in 1948, marked a turning point in the understanding of problems that had plagued communication theory since the advent of electronic communications. Shannon was less concerned with semantics than with the capacity to measure the *quantity* of information transmitted. In its most basic form, information theory represents an effort to define the relation among five elements that make up any communication system: sender, receiver, channel, code, and message. For communication to take place, a human or nonhuman sender must be able to send a coded message across a channel to a receiver who can decipher the transmission. Shannon developed an extraordinarily complex mathematical theory to demonstrate that information can be measured in *quantifiable bits*. The amount of information is inversely proportional to its probability. In other words, the more probable an occurrence or event, the less information it communicates and vice versa. The transmission of messages presupposes the coding of information in a readable form. By providing parameters of constraint, a code or set of codes makes some messages possible and others impossible. Expressed in linguistics terms proposed by Saussure, code is the language (*la langue*) that is the condition of the possibility of the message, which is speech or word (*la parole*). When information theory is combined with the technological capacity to transfer information created by computers, cybernetic systems become networks of communication that are regulated by the orderly flow of information.

Cybernetic theory provides a way to understand mechanical, digital, organic, and bodily systems as well as their interrelationship. Anthony Wilden's concise clarification of this expanded view of communication is helpful.

> All behavior is communication. Communication, by definition, is an attribute of system and involves a structure. Structure concerns frameworks, channels, and coding; system concerns processes, transmissions, and messages. . . . Language includes all the communicational processes and possibilities of less highly organized,

primarily digital, communicational systems, as well as specific linguistic properties. Language is not only a means of communication and behavior; it also imposes specific systemic and structural constraints on the ways in which we perceive and act upon the world and each other.[7]

When organisms are interpreted in terms of language, cybernetics, information, and communications theory, the body appears to be smart rather than dumb meat. Drawing on cybernetic and information theory, feminist critic Donna Haraway explains that "a cyborg is a cybernetic organism, a hybrid of machine and organism, a creature of social reality as well as a creature of fiction. . . . Modern medicine is also full of cyborgs between organism and machine, each conceived as coded devices, in an intimacy and with a power that was not generated in the history of sexuality."[8] Wearing my pancreas on my belt, I am, without a doubt, a cyborg. As Haraway suggests, my condition is not exceptional because in today's wired world we have all become cyborgs.

45

Before turning our attention to a consideration of the microbiotics of information and intelligence in the immune systems of smart bodies, it will be helpful to consider two additional metaphoric frameworks for the interpretation of immunology: military espionage and alien immigration.[9] The most important breakthroughs in molecular biology, genetics, and immunology took place in the decade after the end of the Second World War. Not only technology but also the language in which it was described exercised an enormous influence on postwar scientific research and development. Since the formulation of information theory, philosophers, mathematicians, and scientists have insisted on the relevance of cybernetics for understanding living systems. *In Cybernetics—or Control and Communication in Animal and Machine* (1948), Wiener already argued that an adequate theory of information makes it possible to establish the isomorphism of living and nonliving systems. Such claims remained largely speculative until the remarkable developments in molecular biology in the middle of the century. At the same time that advances in the understanding of the immune system were being made in the 1950s, Watson and Crick were describing their revolutionary discovery of the mechanisms regulating DNA and RNA with terms like *translation, transcription, coding, decoding,* and *cracking the genetic code.* As the tensions of the Cold War increased, militaristic, espionage, and counterespionage rhetoric became widely accepted for describing biological processes.

Australian microbiologist F. Macfarlane Burnet, who was one of the pioneers in what Warwick Anderson and Ian Mackay aptly label "the science of the self," was particularly "fond of notions of control, communication, feedback, coding, message, memory, replication, and pattern" to describe the immune system. In his scientific articles, he politicized these ideas in ways that would eventually become insidious. Anderson and Mackay point out that

> as a biological theorist, Burnet drew on concepts and metaphors circulating during the Cold War. He translated an older militaristic discourse on defense and attack into the new language of control, communication, recognition, tolerance, and surveillance. He emphasized relational

subjectivity and worried about rigid conformity to external models. His immunological manifestos expressed concern about porous boundaries of self and other, and fears of overreaction and hyper-sensitivity. Finely attuned to the American and Australian politics of the Cold War, Burnet intuitively proposed matching metaphors and concepts—figures and tropes that derived from the prevailing thought style.[10]

As these remarks suggest, the scientific literature devoted to the immune system reflects a violence and hostility similar to that expressed in the drawings and puppets children created in the Berrie Center's Pancreas Project. The word *immune* derives from the Latin *immunis*, which means exempt from a public service, burden, or charge; free, exempt. Its use in connection with the investigation of disease and its prevention dates from 1880. Since the middle of the last century, the terms biological and medical researchers have used to characterize immunological processes present a picture of a body engaged in a life-and-death struggle with others who are constantly attacking it. Recalling the image of the ancient physician-philosopher Heraclitus, life is a war and the only guarantee of survival is a good defense system. The immune system is, in effect, a strategic defense initiative (SDI) in which vigilant observers patrol the outer and inner borders of the body to keep out hostile invaders that threaten it. Any adequate defense system requires a sophisticated intelligence community. The complex struggle for recognition between self and other involves an intricate game of espionage in which agents and counteragents (chemical and otherwise) employ elaborate

47

disguises and deceits to dupe their opponents and thereby gain a decisive offensive or defensive advantage. One of the most important ploys in espionage and counterespionage is the ability to trick the enemy by sending false messages that are mistaken for true and true messages that appear to be false. In addition to deceit, defense agents must be able to develop and break codes that convey the messages upon which every SDI depends. When messages are intercepted, interrupted, or misread, the defense system breaks down and the enemy wins.

In her informative book *Flexible Bodies: Tracking Immunity in American Culture from the Days of Polio to the Age of AIDS*, Emily Martin explores the way the military and espionage language used by scientists to describe the immune system spills over into the media and popular culture. She reports that the cover of *Time* magazine on May 23, 1988, carried the headline, "The Battle Inside the Body: New Discoveries Show How the Immune System Fights Disease." Two years later the cover story in *U.S. News and World Report* was entitled "The Body at War: New Breakthroughs in How We Fight Disease." In these articles, the body is described as summoning an army of agents to fend off the threatening horde. Martin points out that in addition to a steady flow of magazines, comics, and popular books using militaristic language and images throughout the 1960s and 1970s, the immune system even played a leading role in the 1966 film *The Fantastic Voyage*, which starred Raquel Welch. When a Russian scientist, who had defected, developed an infection, a team of Americans designed a miniature submarine to travel through the patient's blood vessels. "While wearing a diving suit outside the submarine [inside the patient's bloodstream], Raquel Welch was attacked by antibodies. These were depicted as flickering shapes that adhered tightly to her chest and nearly suffocated her, until, just in the nick of time, the male members of the team managed (more than slightly lasciviously) to pull them off with their hands. In the end, the villain of the drama (a double agent) was horribly killed, suffocated by the billowing white mass of macrophage as the ship passed through a lymph node."[11]

With the end of the Cold War, warfare and espionage rhetoric easily slipped into the paranoid discourse of dangerous aliens and immigrants, who threaten to infect the body politic by slipping across porous borders. Since these aliens supposedly bring filth, contamination, and corruption, it is necessary to develop countermeasures to protect natives from disease. For many of those responsible for homeland security, the best defense against illegal immigration is to build a secure wall and then patrol it with both armed agents and the most sophisticated surveillance technology.

The rhetoric of infection and disease is a two-way street—scientists appropriate the language of politics and technology to describe disease, and philosophers and critics use the language of immunology to describe political developments. With the accelerating spread of globalization, some philosophers have turned to the language of the immune system to describe what is occurring. Anticipating the rise of nationalism and hostility toward immigrants, the controversial German philosopher Peter Sloterdijk uses the language of immunology to compare nascent nationalisms to "classical empires."

It becomes apparent why the attempts of classical meta-physics to conceive all that is as a concentrically organized monosphere were doomed to failure. . . . In fact, such a hyper-orb, because of its forced abstractness, was a flawed immunological design to begin with. The widespread homesickness for the Aristotelian world that is seeing a particular revival today, which recognizes its goal in the word "cosmos" and its longing in the phrase "world soul," exists not least because we do not practice any historical immunology, and draw the dangerously false conclusion from the evident immunodeficiencies of contemporary cultures that earlier world systems were constructed better in this respect.[12]

The escalating rhetoric of alien immigration, infection, and immunity has made the political situation much worse in the two decades since Sloterdijk was writing.

The images and metaphors in all these interpretive frameworks presuppose that the immune system involves an oppositional logic of either/or (0/1), which results in a zero-sum game played between self and nonself. However, when the immune system turns on itself in autoimmune disease, such oppositional logic becomes self-contradictory. For the person suffering from diabetes or any other auto-immune disease, the self is never simply itself but is always also the other of itself, and the other is never sim-ply an enemy or alien but is always at the same time the self itself. The implications of this complicated and strangely inclusive understanding of the self and other are clear in the last metaphor for the immune system—the Intranet. An examination of the biochemistry of the immune system and autoimmunity illuminates the operation of the bodily Intranet.

Smart bodies consist of a network of networks that process information in ways approximating the operation of distributed neural networks in the brain as well as in computational machines outside and sometimes connected to the body. The immune system is a quasi-cognitive network responsible for protecting the health and stability of the organism. In the rhetorical terms I have been considering, the body is constantly engaged in a struggle with biological and chemical agents that are attacking it. The recognition of nonself obviously presupposes the ability to identify oneself. At the most rudimentary level, self-identity and difference from others are not merely a social construct but also a biological or, more precisely, a biochemical fact. This recognition of self-identity is not innate and thus must be learned. Each cell in the body has a protein structure on its surface that identifies it as self. During their developmental process, cells in the immune system learn how to distinguish the body's own protein structure and differentiate it from the protein structure of every alien cell. Self-identity is never secure; therefore, the self must constantly differentiate itself from nonself. The effective operation of the immune system involves coding, messaging, memory, cognition, and interpretation. These functions require the interaction of other agents in networks distributed throughout the body.

In the body's struggle with disease, invaders are antigens, and the defense network is formed by an "army" of lymphocytes, some of which secrete antibodies and some of which attack cellular antigens directly. There are two types of immune response: humoral and cell mediated. Humoral immunity is mediated by large molecules found in fluids outside cells. The cells involved in the immune system are lymphocytes, which are a class of white blood cells. Though all lymphocytes are produced in bone marrow, some migrate to lymphatic tissues and organs and others pass through the thymus gland (located behind the sternum between the lungs), where they undergo further specialization. The former are called B-lymphocytes, which produce the antibodies that are responsible for humoral response, and the latter T-lymphocytes, which are responsible for cell-mediated response.

Millions of foreign agents seek to cross the body's porous borders. These hostile invaders are marked by antigens that bear a unique identity formed by specific molecules on their surface. This protein structure constitutes a code that must be deciphered by the body's defense system. One of the major breakthroughs in immunology was Niels Jerne's discovery in 1954 that the human body is programmed to detect and to respond to an astonishing one hundred million or more antigens. Jerne arrived at his momentous insight while walking home from the Danish State Serum Institute in Copenhagen. Ten years later he described his discovery in philosophical terms he borrowed from Søren Kierkegaard.

> "Can the truth (*the capability to synthesize an antibody*) be learned? If so, it must be assumed not to pre-exist; to be learned, it must be acquired. We are thus confronted with the difficulty to which Socrates calls attention in the *Meno*, namely that it makes as little sense to search for what one

does not know as to search for what one knows; what one knows one cannot search for, since one knows it already, and what one does not know one cannot search for, since one does not even know what to search for. Socrates resolves this difficulty by postulating that learning is nothing but recollection. The truth (*the capability to synthesize an antibody*) cannot be brought in, but was already immanent."

The above paragraph is a translation of the first lines of Søren Kierkegaard's *Philosophical Fragments*. By replacing the word "truth" by the italicized words, the statement can be made to present the logical basis of the selective theories of antibody formation. Or, in the parlance of Molecular Biology, synthetic potentialities cannot be imposed upon nucleic acid, but must pre-exist.[13]

53

According to Jerne's natural selection theory, the body randomly produces antibodies capable of recognizing virtually every possible antigen it might encounter. Each person's set of antibodies differs because the underlying gene arrangements that give rise to so many different antibody genes is random. The revolutionary aspect of Jerne's theory is his contention that the antibodies are produced in the absence of antigens. In other words, the body is preprogrammed for possible future battles *before* the so-called enemy appears. F. M. Burnet refined Jerne's analysis to form the clonal selection theory, which specifies the precise recognition mechanisms at work in the immune system.

The strategies for recognizing antigens are somewhat different in the humoral and cell-mediated response. In the humoral response, a specific antibody produced by a

B-lymphocyte and present as a receptor on the surface of the lymphocyte recognizes a limited range of antigens and responds by producing more antibodies, which are released into the blood stream to combat the infection. The recognition mechanism in B-lymphocytes is similar to a digital function in which the decoding of a message turns on a switch that sets in motion antibody production. The antigen-antibody dyad forms something like a lock-key structure with part of the surface structure of the antigen, the epitope (mentioned earlier), serving as a lock that can be opened by a customized key. The keylike part of the antibody is a protein structure that fits the antigen epitope. Since there are at least one hundred million antibodies in the human body, the sorting process necessary for an effective response to the presence of aliens is extraordinarily complex. When the key fits the lock (that is, when the binary molecular structures unite), proper identification and the immune response begin.

This process of recognition can be described in different terms. The antibody must *read* the message or *decode* the program of the antigen. Once the antibody *understands* exactly what the antigen is *saying*, it *knows* how to respond. The response of the body is twofold. First, the antibody's recognition of the antigen as a foreign agent triggers the production of more antibodies by B-lymphocytes to ward off the invasion. According to Burnet's clonal selection theory, the lymphocyte clones itself, thereby producing additional lymphocytes, which make the same antibody. These antibodies are released into the bloodstream and circulate to neutralize or destroy antigens. One of the most remarkable features of the immune system is that some of the cloned

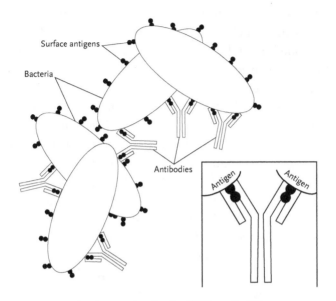

FIGURE 2.1 Antigen—Antibody. William DeWitt.

lymphocytes are brought to the brink of response (that is, brought to the stage where they are capable of producing antibodies) and then deactivated. These antibodies form something like an army of reserves that constitute the organism's *immunological memory*. When the body is attacked again by the same antigen, the deactivated recruits are called to active duty. Having already undergone extensive training, the activated reserves can respond quickly and effectively when ordered to do so. This mechanism explains why, in some cases, a person who has had a disease once is immunized against further occurrences of the illness.

T-lymphocytes are more complex than B-lymphocytes. There are three basic types of T-cells: regulatory T-cells, which suppress or turn on antibody production; suppressor T-cells, which turn off antibody production when an adequate humoral response has been achieved; and killer T-cells, which attack invading or infected cells directly. These cells also react hostilely to implants and transplanted organs. In order to decipher the code of the antigen, killer T-cells need the assistance of cells in the blood known as macrophages, which are large cells that serve as scavengers that engulf microbes and devour dead or damaged cells as well as cellular debris. The antigen cannot be recognized as nonself until a macrophage consumes the foreign microbe and presents it to the killer T-cell. After ingesting the alien invader, the macrophage places the portion of the protein structure (the epitope) that defines the antigen on its own surface. The killer T-cell decodes the antigen unless the foreign protein structure is presented along with a molecular trace of the body's own self-identity. When the macrophage presents the antigen, it is placed beside the cellular signature of the body in a way that enables the killer T-cell to distinguish self and nonself. The recognition of the antigen by the killer T-cell follows the lock-and-key pattern of B-lymphocytes. The macrophage releases a hormonelike molecule of interleukin, which causes the killer T-cell to divide and form an "army of defense agents." Fortified T-cells attack the antigen by secreting a protein that pierces the membrane of the alien cell and releases fluids that eventually kill the cell.

Self vs. Other . . . Identity vs. Difference. This immunological process is a biological version of what Hegel describes in his famous account of the master-slave relationship as "the struggle for recognition." When the immune system works, it functions as a secure wall constructed to keep out illegal aliens. Beta cells and the three types of T-cells serve as border agents that keep the body safe by patrolling the wall and turning away undesirables with devastating diseases.

Sometimes, however, the immune system does not work, or, even worse, it malfunctions and betrays the body it is supposed to protect by attacking the self as if it were an other. Whereas in proper immune response self and other are clearly differentiated, autoimmune diseases reveal that the self is, paradoxically, simultaneously itself and the other of itself. When the cells that are supposed to target invaders attack the self, the result is self-destruction by self-consumption. Haraway correctly observes that "we seem invaded not just by threatening 'non-selves' that the immune system guards against, but more fundamentally by our own strange parts. No wonder autoimmune disease carries such awful significance, marked from the first suspicion of its existence in 1901 by [Julius] Morgenroth and [Paul] Ehrlich's term, *horror autotoxicus*."[14] During the past century, scientists confirmed the suspicions of Morgenroth and Erlich many times over. In every case of *autotoxicus*, the disease is caused by a malfunction of the immune system. Scientists are now convinced that autoimmune diseases are caused by a miseducation of cells that leads to a breakdown in the communications networks in the body. During their educational process, B-cells are exposed to self proteins, and if any of their antibodies bind tightly to them at this stage of development, the B-cell self-destructs. But sometimes cells that mistake self for other escape into the blood or lymph system, where they can circulate for years. In some

57

people, these killer T-cells are activated and target cells in specific organs of the body. Scientists still do not understand what triggers this process.

The pancreas is part of the endocrine system, which also includes the pituitary, pineal, thyroid, and adrenal glands, as well as ovaries and testes. All these glands are ductless and, in cooperation with the nervous system, regulate bodily activities by secreting hormones into the blood. Within the decentered information networks of the body, responsibility for short-term adjustments is delegated to the nervous system and long-term regulation of bodily functions is controlled by the endocrine system. Endocrine glands operate like cybernetic systems that sustain the metabolic homeostasis necessary for the stability of the organism. The resulting homeostasis breaks down when the cells that are supposed to protect the body mistakenly attack the insulin-producing cells in the pancreas. Protecting the body at the most rudimentary level is made more difficult by a strange phenomenon known as "molecular mimicry." Molecules create disguises, which add layers of deceit and duplicity to the intelligence and counterintelligence drama played out along the body's internal and external borders. Irun Cohen describes possible complications in the body's response to antigens.

> The challenge is compounded by the fact that the self and the invader are made up of the same building blocks: proteins, carbohydrates, nucleic acids, and lipids. What is more, molecules such as enzymes or hormones that perform key biological functions tend to be conserved in evolution so that the self and invader may have

identical—or at least very similar—molecules. Finally, it seems that some pathogens actually make hostlike antigens as a means of disguise. . . . It appears that antigenic "mimicry" is a persistent feature of the struggle between self and pathogen.[15]

Once the body turns against itself, it may lack the resources to turn off the process of self-destruction.

While there still is no cure for type 1 diabetes, promising research is being done that points toward several different, though related, approaches. Given the success of organ transplants to treat other diseases, the most obvious solution might seem to be to transplant the pancreas from another person or perhaps even from an animal. In an effort to address the persistent difficulty of an adequate supply of human organs, experiments are being conducted to determine whether it would be possible to clone pigs whose pancreases could be transplanted in people. Such cross-species grafting is known as xenotransplantation. This procedure obviously would require tissue compatibility between human and animals as well as developing a way to prevent the rejection of the alien organ. The latter problem is especially acute for diabetics because the immunosuppressant drugs necessary for transplant recipients further weaken their already-compromised immune systems and make patients extremely vulnerable to dangerous infections. While pancreatic transplants have not yet been tried in humans, pig pancreases have been transplanted in monkeys.

The difficulties with whole-organ transplants has led other researchers to investigate the possibility of transplanting only the insulin-producing cells of the pancreas. This approach creates the possibility of addressing the two primary problems with pancreas transplants. First, the likelihood of rejection might be overcome by encapsulating beta cells in a protective membrane that would let vital fluids out but not allow killer T-cells in. Second, it might be possible to overcome the problem of cell supply by educating stem cells to become insulin-producing beta cells that are self-tolerant. It would also be necessary to figure out a way to turn off the switch that transforms some lymphocytes into killer T-cells that attack the body they are supposed to protect. This method has been successful in mice, and experiments with human cells drawn from the skin are now underway. The cells would have to be trained not to attack the body's insulin-producing cells without inhibiting the immune response so much that the body's defense system would become ineffective. Every kind of transplant or implant further complicates the self-nonself relation and further confounds oppositions like inside/outside and natural/artificial. This hybridity discloses an alternative structure of bodily being. Clinical trials that use stem cells from a person's skin are nearing approval. If any of these solutions were to work, type 1 diabetes would be cured and the need for costly and onerous therapies requiring insulin, syringes, monitors, and pumps would no longer be necessary. In addition to solving the mysteries of the immune system, the challenges scientists face are compounded by financial difficulties. With university funds for research dwindling, corporate support becomes more important, but since diabetes is so lucrative, many pharmaceutical companies are ambivalent about finding a cure and are thus reluctant at times to provide adequate support.

These therapies simultaneously mimic and reverse the dynamics of autoimmunity. While immune reactions presuppose the logic of noncontradiction (*either* self *or* nonself), autoimmune diseases involve the paradoxical logic (both/and) in which the self is *both* itself *and* the other of itself. Far from an aberrant condition, *autoimmunity discloses our shared condition.* Jacques Derrida makes this point in his book *Specters of Marx.*

> The living ego is auto-immune. . . . To protect its life, to constitute itself as unique living ego, to relate as the same, to itself, it is necessarily led to welcome the other within (so many figures of death [and disease]: differ*a*nce of the technical apparatus, iterability, non-uniqueness, prosthesis, synthetic image, simulacrum, all of which begins with language, before language), it must therefore take the immune defenses apparently meant for the non-ego, the enemy, the opposite, the adversary and direct them at once *for itself and against itself.*[16]

61

Derrida's language is convoluted, but his point is clear. Insofar as the self establishes its identity by its difference from others (that is, nonself), the nonself is the condition of the possibility of the identity of the self. The self is, therefore, forever haunted by an otherness that inevitably renders it spectral. In different terms, the outside is not merely outside, but is always already within as an interior exterior that simultaneously divides the self from itself and connects it to nonself. This interplay of self and nonself begins at the biochemical and bodily level and extends to social, political, and technological processes from which the self is never separated. No one has done more to complicate and enrich the dynamics of identity and difference than Derrida. However, his suspicions about technology, which he shares with Heidegger, prevent him from extending his analysis to include the expanding technological matrix in which we are entangled.

The careful consideration of the specific biochemical operation of autoimmune disease points to the sixth and, for now, final metaphorical framework for understanding bodily being. The body is an Intranet, which is a network of multiple contending and cooperating networks. I have considered only one type of disease in relation to one primary organ. The pancreas, as we have seen, is part of the endocrine system, with multiple interrelated organs that are connected to every other organ and system in the body. The structure of all these networks is fractal—that is to say, they have the same structure at every level from the cellular to the organism as a whole. Like other accounts of immunity and autoimmunity, the notion of the Intranet obviously reflects the technologies of its time. If the either/or language of warfare and espionage appropriates terms drawn from the Cold War, the idea of the body as an Intranet mirrors the language of the Internet era. When the Cold War seemed to end with the collapse of the Soviet Union, many people believed that there had been a transition from a world of walls that separate to a world of networks and webs that connect. Emerging information, communications, and network technologies, which led to the end of the Cold War, provided rich metaphors for what emerged in its wake. Revolutionary changes did not occur with the invention of mainframe computers in the 1940s, 1950s, and 1960s, or even with the introduction of personal computers in the 1970s; rather, the seismic shift occurred when high-speed computers, personal computers, mobile devices, and data banks were connected first locally in Intranets during the 1980s, and then globally through the Internet during the 1990s and after.

While these developments were unfolding, two events marked a shift in our understanding of the immune system: first, the 1970 publication of Jerne's important paper, bearing the suggestive title "Towards a Network Theory of the Immune System," and, second, the scientific investigation of emergent complex systems and networks. In what was initially presented as a talk at the Basel Institute for Immunology, Jerne begins by summarizing developments in the understanding of the immune system from 1950 to 1970 before proceeding to make predictions about what he believes will be the major theoretical developments from 1970 to 1990. After proposing a series of terminological changes, he makes his central point. "The immune system displays a number of *dualisms*. The first of these is the occurrence of T lymphocytes and B lymphocytes with partly synergic, partly antagonistic interactions. The second dualism is . . . that antibody molecules must recognize as well as be recognized. These properties lead to the establishment of a *network* [emphasis added], and as antibody molecules occur both free and as receptor molecules on lymphocytes, this network intertwines with cells and molecules."[17] Jerne's point is that the immune system consists of multiple binary oppositions whose interactions create a communications *network* in which coded signals in the form of protein structures on the surface of molecules form messages sent and received among internal and external agents. Health and disease depend on the accurate processing of this information.

In describing the immune system as a network, Jerne draws a direct comparison with the nervous system. It is worth quoting his argument at length because it both summarizes my analysis in this chapter and points to the account of different aspects of the Internet in the next two chapters.

> In finishing, I should only like to point out that the immune system, when viewed as a functional network dominated by a mainly suppressive Eigen [Self]—behavior, but open to stimuli from the outside, bears a striking resemblance to the nervous system. These two systems stand out among all other organs of our body by their ability to respond adequately to an enormous variety of signals. Both systems display dichotomies and dualisms. The cells of both systems can receive as well as transmit signals. In both systems the signals can be either excitatory or inhibitory. . . . The nervous system is a network of neurons in which the axon and the dendrites of one nerve cell form synaptic connections with sets of other nerve cells. In the human body there are about 10^{13} lymphocytes as compared to 10^{10} nerve cells. Lymphocytes do not need connections by fibers in order to form a network. As lymphocytes can move freely, they can interact either by direct encounters or through the antibody molecules they release. The network resides in the ability of these elements to recognize as well as to be recognized. Like for the nervous system, the modulation of the network by

foreign signals represents its adaptation to the outside world. Early imprints leave the deepest traces. Both systems thereby learn from experience and build up a memory by reinforcement and that is deposited in persistent network interactions that cannot be transmitted to our offspring.[18]

Recognition of the similarities between the network structure of the nervous system and the immune system makes the long-standing opposition between mind and body obsolete. Mind is always embodied and body is always intelligent—both in themselves and in their inextricable interrelationship, they form distributed cognitive networks.

65

In the years following the publication of Jerne's network theory of the immune system, there was growing interest in the study of complex systems. Researchers in a variety of fields identified common patterns in physical, biological, social, political, economic, cultural, and technological networks. In 1984, the Santa Fe Institute was established to promote interdisciplinary research in complexity theory. Three years later, the institute published a volume entitled *Theoretical Immunology*, which includes an important article by Francisco Varela and his colleagues, entitled "Cognitive Networks: Immune, Neural, and Otherwise," in which they extend Jerne's theory by interpreting it in terms of emergent complex adaptive networks.[19] They refine Jerne's argument about the similarity between the immune system and the nervous system by drawing a distinction between the interpretation of cognition as a symbolic process and connectionist models of cognition.

The study of biological and artificial cognitive mechanisms was heavily marked by the tradition that considered any form of knowledge as necessarily linked to symbols and rules, in the tradition of logic. This gave rise to
the *symbolic* paradigm, where cognition is identified with
information processing: rule-based manipulation of
symbols. After many years of work with this symbolic
paradigm, especially in neuroscience and artificial intelligence, it has become clear that such mechanisms are far
too brittle, too inflexible to approach living expertise.

The alternative view, revived recently from initial ideas
dating back to the 1950s, is usually referred to as *connectionism*. Basically, the idea is to leave symbols aside and to
start any analysis (or construction) from simple computing elements, each one carrying some value of activation
which is calculated on the basis of other elements in the
network through a dynamical rule. . . . We will argue here
that immune networks share with connectionist ideas
the distributed dynamical base. . . .

A key idea of a network perspective is that the on-going
activity of units, together with constraints from the system's surroundings, constantly produces *emerging* global
patterns over the entire network which constitutes its performance. The network itself decides how to tune its
component elements in mutual relationships that give the
entire system a capacity (recognition, memory, etc.), which
is not available to components in isolation.[20]

The interpretation of the immune system as an emerging
complex adaptive network suggests the way the body
extends beyond its apparent borders and becomes a node

in recursive worldwide webs. The Intranet of the body, which forms the infrastructure of its functions, does not stand alone but is wired in dynamic feedback and feed-forward loops to the intervolving Internet of Things and Internet of Bodies.

3

Internet of Things

Two games: Chess and Go. Two films: *The Man vs. the Machine* and *AlphaGo*. Two types of artificial intelligence: symbolic AI and connectionist AI.

On February 10, 1996, Garry Kasparov played IBM's Deep Blue in a highly touted match in Philadelphia. The cover of *Newsweek* had a picture of Kasparov with the headline warning "The Brain's Last Stand." Charles Osgood, anchor of the CBS evening news, solemnly warned, "forget the hundreds of thousands of dollars, the future of humanity is on the line." Initially, it seemed that the machine would triumph over the human—Deep Blue won the first game. But Kasparov rallied and won three and tied two of the remaining games. A year later, there was a rematch in which Kasparov won the first game, and Deep Blue won the second. After three draws, Deep Blue won the decisive sixth game and became the first computer to defeat a world champion in a multiple-game match. Geneticist and digital medicine researcher Eric Topol reports that, shortly after he had lost the match, Kasparov wrote that "he thought he could sense 'a new kind of intelligence across the table.' He recalled, 'The scrum of photographers around the table doesn't annoy a computer. There is no looking into your opponent's eyes to read his mood, or seeing if his hand hesitates a little above the clock, indicating a lack of confidence. As a believer in chess as a form of psychological, and not just intellectual, warfare, playing against something with no psyche was troubling from the start.' "[1]

With this unprecedented match, the question of the relation of machine intelligence and human intelligence became urgent. As early as 1948, Alan Turing published a paper titled "Intelligent Machinery, a Heretical Theory," in which he emphatically asserted, "My contention is that machines can be constructed which will simulate the behavior of the human mind very closely." To support his claim, he takes the example of playing two games—chess and Go. The machine Turing imagines would have a typewriter or keyboard to input information and a memory to store all the moves that had been made in any game it had played. It would also be possible to record other moves that could have been made. Eventually, the machine would take a self-reflexive turn by remembering the moves it makes and developing ways to sort through its stored knowledge. Having defined these parts, Turing proceeds to explain how the machine would work. "New forms of index might be introduced on account of special features observed in the indexes already used. The indexes would be used in this sort of way. Whenever a choice has to be made as to what to do next, features of the present situation are looked up in the indexes available, and the previous choice in similar situations, and the outcome, good or bad, is discovered." Turing is not only confident that such a machine can be built, but goes so far as to predict that "it seems probable that it would not take long to outstrip our feeble powers. There would be no question of the machines dying, and they would be able to converse with each other to sharpen their wits."[2]

The abstract computational machine Turing describes became a model for early computers. In a paper published two years later (1950), titled "Computing Machinery and Intelligence," he outlines the principles of what became the standard form of artificial intelligence for two decades. Symbolic artificial intelligence came to be known as Good Old Fashioned Artificial Intelligence (GOFAI). "The idea behind digital computers may be explained by saying that these machines are intended to carry out any operations which could be done by a human computer. The human computer is supposed to be following fixed rules; he has no authority to deviate from them in any detail. We may suppose that these rules are supplied in a book, which is altered whenever he is put on to a new job. He has also an unlimited supply of paper on which he does his calculations. He may also do his multiplications and additions on a 'desk machine,' but this is not important."[3] In this computational model, the problem being analyzed must be broken down and represented mathematically, logically, or symbolically. These representations must then be coded digitally. Codes and coding have become so much a part of our lives that it is easy to overlook their far-reaching presuppositions and implications. Code, as Katherine Hayles argues, has become something like an "unconscious language."[4] The digital opposition between 0 and 1 mirrors the binary opposition

Saussure identifies with the structure of language (*la langue*) that is the underlying condition of speech (*la parole*). This isomorphism makes it possible to translate language into code and code into language. In his widely acclaimed novel, *Book of Numbers*, Joshua Cohen clarifies the relationship between code and language. "Binary code—an encryption that's simultaneously a translation, in how it renders two different systems compatible, equitable. 'Bits'—the term itself is a contradiction ('binary digits')—are the fundamentals of any expression: not just of integers but also of language, and so of instructions, commands."[5] So understood, machine and mind meet in code.

72

As our consideration of the immune system and autoimmune disease has shown, the efficacy of code extends beyond mental operation to bodily and even biochemical processes. With Watson's and Crick's cracking of the genetic code, it became clear that life itself is programmed. At the University of Paris, former director of the Institute of the History of Science and Technology Georges Canguilhem explains the seismic shift involved in the discovery of how genetic information or code determines the way cells synthesize the building blocks of protein for new cells.

> In changing the scale on which the characteristic phenomena of life—which is to say, the structuration of matter and the regulation of functions, including the structuration of function—are studied, contemporary biology has also adopted a new language. It has dropped the vocabulary and concepts of classical mechanics, physics and chemistry, all more or less directly based on geometrical models, in favor of the vocabulary of linguistics and

communications theory. Messages, information, programs, code, instructions, decoding: these are the new concepts in the life sciences.[6]

Biological heredity, like the immune system, entails communication and, on occasion, miscommunication, which can lead to mutations that create new forms of life or diseases that lead to death. The ubiquity of coded information extends the interoperability of machines from minds to bodies.

Code is a necessary but not a sufficient condition of machine intelligence. In addition to accumulating and storing coded information, in Good Old Fashioned Artificial Intelligence machines must be given instructions for how to process this information. Turing writes, "We have mentioned that the 'book of rules' supplied to the computer is replaced in the machine by a part of the store. It is then called the 'table of instructions.' It is the duty of the control to see that these instructions are obeyed correctly and in the right order. The control is so constructed that this necessarily happens. . . . Constructing instruction tables is usually described as 'programming.' To 'program a machine to carry out the operation A' means to put the appropriate instruction table into the machine so that it will do A."[7]

This book of rules is made up of algorithms. The word *algorithm* derives from the name of Algorithmi, who was a Persian mathematician, astronomer, and geographer. In the twelfth century, his Arabic treatises *Hindu-Arabic Numeral System* and *Algebra* were translated into Latin, and during the Middle Ages al-Gorithm was the most widely read

73

mathematician in Europe. "Algorithm" did not acquire its current meaning until the late nineteenth century. An algorithm is a precise set of instructions for a computer to carry out procedures necessary to solve a specific problem. Algorithms are what give computers the agency through which they not only communicate with other machines but also have a transformative effect on minds, bodies, and even the world. Yuval Noah Harari goes so far as to claim that "'algorithm' is arguably the single most important concept in our world."[8]

With this understanding of symbolic artificial intelligence and its implementation in computers, let us return to the game of chess. The possibility of inventing a machine that can play chess has long captured the imagination of creative thinkers and writers. In 1769, the Hungarian nobleman Wolfgang von Kempelen claimed to have created an automaton named The Turk that could play chess. This invention appeared to be an upgrade of the automatons designed several decades earlier by the French artist Jacques de Vaucanson, whose mechanical devices were the precursors of today's robots. Vaucanson's constructions included the Tambourine Player and the Flute Player, which was a life-sized figure that could play twelve songs. His most sensational automaton was his Digesting Duck, which consisted of more than four hundred moving parts. The duck could flap its wings, drink water, eat grain, and even defecate. Von Kempelen's chess player seemed to improve on Vaucanson's machines by adding cognitive processes to its repertoire, but was exposed as a fake that concealed a person inside the machine who moved the pieces on the board. These automatons created a sensation throughout Europe and sparked lively debates about the relationship between humans and machines that provoked discussions about the defining characteristics of human and what came to be known as artificial intelligence. After von Kempelen's death, Johann Nepomuk Maelzel took The Turk on a European tour, and in 1825 he brought the automaton to the United States. Maelzel's roadshow had all the glitz and intrigue of a Penn & Teller magic performance.

Edgar Allan Poe was intrigued by The Turk and wrote a long essay, "Maelzel's Chess Player" (1836), in which he exposes The Turk as a fraud in seventeen numbered and carefully argued steps. Poe's suspicion is clear from the outset.

—

> Wherever seen it has been an object of intense curiosity, to all persons who think. Yet the question of the *modus operandi*—is still undetermined. Nothing has been written on this topic which can be considered as decisive—and accordingly we find everywhere men of mechanical genius, of great general astuteness, and discriminative understanding, who make no scruple in pronouncing the Automaton a *pure machine*, unconnected with human agency in its movements, and consequently, beyond all comparison, the most astonishing of the inventions of mankind. And such it would undoubtedly be, were they right in their supposition.[9]

After briefly describing earlier magic shows as well as Vaucanson's duck, Poe compares The Turk unfavorably to Charles Babbage's Analytic Machine and proceeds to lay out the requirement for genuine machine intelligence.[10]

Arithmetical or algebraical calculations are, from their very nature, fixed and determinate. Certain *data* being given, certain results necessarily and inevitably follow. These results have dependence upon nothing, and are influenced by nothing but the *data* originally given. And the question to be solved proceeds, or should proceed, to a final determination, by a succession of unerring steps liable to no change, and subject to no modification. This being the case, we can without difficulty conceive the *possibility* of so arranging a piece of mechanism, that upon starting it in accordance with the *data* of the question to be solved, it should continue its movements regularly, progressively, and undeviatingly towards the required solution, since these movements, however complex, are never imagined to be otherwise than finite and determinate.[11]

76

Convinced that The Turk does not meet these requirements, Poe exposes the man in the machine. In developing his argument about the automaton, he was actually describing what became his signature analytic method in his detective stories. When placed in a longer historical perspective, Poe's requirements for a thinking machine anticipate both the era of Big Data and the foundational principles of Good Old Fashioned Artificial Intelligence.

Turing knew Poe's essay and recognized its importance. He begins a paper entitled "Digital Computers Applied to Games" (1953) by citing Poe's essay and summarizing previous machines designed to play chess. Turing admits that these efforts have not been very successful and were actually better suited to carnival tents than to scientific laboratories. Nonetheless, he remains convinced that it is possible to build such a machine and defines its conditions. "If one can explain quite unambiguously in English, with the aid of mathematical symbols if required, how a calculation can be done, then it is always possible to program any digital computer to do that calculation, provided the storage capacity is adequate."[12] Turing devotes the rest of his paper to a detailed explanation of how to program a digital computer to play chess. It took more than three decades for Turing's idea to become a reality.

Deep Blue is a direct descendent of von Kempelen's automaton, Poe's "tales of ratiocination" in which the mind functions like a machine, and Turing's mathematical theories about a chess-playing machine. As Freud explains in his classic essay "The Uncanny" ("Das Unheimliche"), there is something strangely disturbing about seemingly intelligent machines. We have seen that Kasparov was unsettled by the computer's lack of affect and its psychological vacuity. He realized that he was competing against a disembodied intelligence devoid of emotion. Turing's conception of machine intelligence implemented in Deep Blue is one of the most radical expressions of the dualism plaguing Western philosophy from Plato to Descartes, in which minds are omnicompetent and bodies are regarded as dumb rather than smart. But when mind is abstracted from its material substrate, serious distortions result. Cognitive science compounds this philosophical mistake by interpreting the mind according to the model of a digital computer operating by the rules of symbolic artificial intelligence. Edwin Hutchins offers a helpful corrective to this influential line of analysis when he argues, "The model of human intelligence as abstract symbol manipulation and the substitution of a mechanized formal symbol-manipulation system for the brain result in the widespread notion in contemporary cognitive science that symbols are inside the head. . . . This mistake has consequences. Why did all the sensorimotor apparatus fall off the person when the computer replaced the brain? It fell off because the computer was never a model of the person to begin with. Remember when the symbols were outside, and the apparatus that fell off is exactly the apparatus that supported interaction with those symbols. When the symbols were put inside, there was no need for eyes, ears, or hands. . . . AI was producing 'deaf, dumb, and blind, paraplegic agents.' "[13]

To get mind back into body and body back into mind, a different kind of artificial intelligence is required. Turing realized this problem and pointed toward an alternative approach when he acknowledged that, to realize their full potential, computers would have to learn how to learn. He makes this point citing a text by one of the most important, fascinating, and overlooked people in the early history of computers—Ada Lovelace, who was the only legitimate child of the great British poet Lord Byron.

Our most detailed information of Babbage's Analytical Engine comes from a memoir by Lady Lovelace (1842). In it she states, "The Analytical Engine has no pretensions to *originate* anything. It can do *whatever we know how to order it to perform.*" This statement is quoted by [Douglas] Hartree (1949) who adds: "This does not imply that it may not be possible to construct electronic equipment which will 'think for itself,' or in which, in biological terms, one could set up a conditioned reflex, which would serve as a basis for 'learning.' " Whether this is possible in principle or not is a stimulating and exciting question, suggested by some of these recent developments. But it did not seem that the machines constructed or projected at the time had this property."[14]

Babbage, regarded by many as the "father of the computer," invented the mechanical computer, which had all the components of today's electronic computers.[15] He named his first computer the "Difference Engine" (1822), which he claimed could "generate mathematical tables of many kinds by the 'method of differences.' "[16] Before Babbage finished building this machine, he became obsessed with designing and constructing a more complex machine modeled after the card-operated Jacquard loom. This remarkable device used punch cards to control looms that created extremely complex woven designs in fabrics. The Analytical Engine (1833) was to be built from thousands of cylinders with interlocking gears, which were to be controlled by a *program* recorded on punched cards, and would include a "store," memory, and a "mill" (CPU). Babbage's friend and collaborator, Ada Lovelace, was arguably the world's first computer programmer.

In many ways, Deep Blue was little more than an electronic version of Babbage's Analytic Machine. In the match with Kasparov, the then state-of-the-art computer used Good Old Fashioned Artificial Intelligence, which functioned as something like a punched card controlling the moves of the pieces on the chessboard. The machine was given a set of rules or instructions and was provided with data from more than 700,000 grandmaster games. Using these rules to search the games, Deep Blue could evaluate 200 million possible positions per second before deciding what move to make. The rules by which the computer processed data and executed decisions were externally derived and did not change. This system, in other words, is hardwired or, in philosophical terms, operates according to a priori principles.

The question Ada Lovelace asked about machine learning raises problems for the machine Turing envisioned. "A better variant of the objection," Turing admits, "says that a machine can never 'take us by surprise.' This statement is a more direct challenge and can be met directly. Machines surprise us with great frequency. This is largely because I do not do a calculation in a hurried, slipshod fashion, taking risks."[17] This response is misguided because the computer does not really do anything new or unexpected. The observer is surprised because of the inadequacy of his or her information or knowledge, not because something truly novel occurs. For machines to learn in ways that would make possible adaptability and creativity that approximate human intelligence, it is necessary to move beyond symbolic artificial intelligence. Turing concludes his important paper by pointing to a future that has become our present.

> We may hope that machines will eventually compete with men in all purely intellectual fields. But which are the best ones to start with? Even this is a difficult decision. Many people think that a very abstract activity, like the playing of chess, would be best. It can also be maintained that it is best to provide the machine with the best sense organs that money can buy, and then teach it to understand and

speak English. This process could follow the normal teaching of a child. Things would be pointed out and named, etc. Again, I do not know what is the right answer, but I think both approaches should be tried.[18]

For this future to become a reality, machines would have to learn how to play Go as well as chess.

Go is an ancient game invented in China around 3,000 years ago that is vastly more complicated and much more popular than chess. Most of the estimated 46 million people who play Go live in Asia. In contrast to chess, which is played on an 8 x 8 grid with 64 spaces, the board for Go is a 19 x 19 grid with 361 spaces. The purpose of the game is to surround more territory than your opponent by placing black or white stones on vacant intersections called "points." The game continues until neither player can make another move. The winner is the player who has surrounded the most territory and has captured more of his or her opponent's stones. It is difficult to comprehend the complexity of Go—the number of Go positions is "$2.081681994 \times 10^{170}$, which is two hundred quinquinquagintillion—and vastly more than the number of the atoms in the universe, which is why it was a much more interesting challenge than a game like checkers or chess."[19] The exceeding complexity of Go makes it extraordinarily difficult to create a machine that can successfully play the game. Meeting this challenge with traditional artificial intelligence proved to be impossible.

As early as 1943, Walter Pitts, a logician working in the area of computational neuroscience, and Warren McCulloch, a neurophysiologist and cybernetician, published a seminal paper, "A Logical Calculus of Ideas Immanent in

Nervous Activity," in which they proposed to model a computer on the structure and operation of the brain. Pitts and McCulloch were the first to suggest a mathematical model of a neural network. While this theory eventually would prove revolutionary, neural networks would not have become the infrastructure of machine learning without the essential contribution of Canadian neurophysiologist Donald Hebb's *The Origin of Behavior* (1949). Hebb invented a learning algorithm based on the dynamics of biological systems that, in principle, could be used in neural networks to create an autonomous learning machine like the one Turing envisioned. The basic principle was that learning alters synaptic connections, thereby changing the wiring of the brain. If there were a way to mimic this process in the nodes of an artificial neural network, machines would be able to learn. Neural networks offered a completely different approach than traditional AI. Though this alternative seemed promising to many computer scientists, it met with widespread skepticism among AI researchers. In 1969, Marvin Minsky and Seymour Papert published *Perceptrons: An Introduction to Computational Geometry,* in which they argued that neural networks were theoretically and practically untenable. This argument changed the direction of AI research for more than twenty years. Symbolic AI displaced neural network theory, leading to what many critics would later call an "artificial intelligence winter."

This winter did not break until the 1980s. With the introduction of high-speed networked computers, neural networks became not only practically viable but were actually preferable for solving many of the most difficult problems. I will consider the structure and operation of neural networks in more detail in what is to follow. Here, it is only necessary to understand that neural networks consist of multiple nodes with multiple connections that form a massive interactive network operating on parallel distributed processing machines. While symbolic AI follows a top-down procedure in which data are processed according to rules that have been input, neural networks have a bottom-up structure. Instead of specific rules or procedures, the machine is given a goal and fed massive amounts of data that it analyzes in recursive processes to find patterns that lead to a possible solution. Seventy-five years after Pitts and McCulloch proposed neural networks and Turing predicted machine learning, the arrival of deep learning was marked when Geoffrey Hinton, Yann LeCun, and Yoshua Bengio received the A. M. Turing Award, which is the Nobel Prize in computing, for their groundbreaking work on neural networks in the 1980s.

83

Neural network theory is also known as connectionism. According to connectionist theory, all mental phenomena are the result of a massive interactive network on which different processes run simultaneously. The circles represent nodes and the lines in figures 3.1 and 3.2 represent their connections. The efficacy of artificial neural networks can be increased by superimposing multiple layers of interconnected nodes.

Input data are processed according to different algorithms—each node reads its input and transmits a signal to other nodes. Hebbian learning is implemented by assigning different weights expressed as numerical values to different inputs and outputs. If the sum total of the weights exceeds a determined threshold value of the

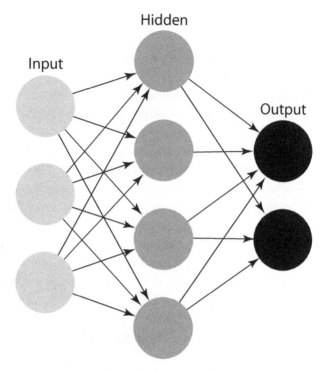

FIGURE 3.1 Single-layer neural network.

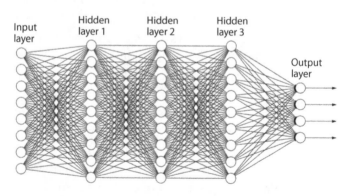

FIGURE 3.2 Deep neural network.

synapse, the neuron fires and activates other neurons; if it is below the threshold, the neuron does not fire and the signal is not transmitted. The firing of the neuron reinforces the strength of the synaptic connection and increases the probability of firing subsequently in similar circumstances. In Hebb's memorable phrase, "neurons that fire together wire together." This coordinated firing reconfigures the network by increasing or decreasing the assigned weight of the connection. These changes are stored and become the memory that makes learning possible.

In his book *The Symbolic Species: The Co-evolution of Language and the Brain,* Terrence Deacon explains,

> What makes the behavior of such nets interesting, and similar to their biological counterparts, is that they can be set up so that all connections between nodes can be modified with respect to their correlation to certain input-output patterns. If individual "connection strengths" can be adjusted to weaken or strengthen the effect of one node on another, the net's behavior can be progressively adapted to fit a given rule linking input patterns to output patterns. This is the analogue to training and learning. There is an almost unlimited range of possible strategies for organizing and training nets. All share the common logic of modifying the local connection with respect to some index of global behavior. Over the course of many trials with many inputs, the performance of a net can thus be trained to converge on a given target set of input-output relationships.[20]

This learning process can be either supervised (semi-autonomous) in which human agents intervene, or

unsupervised (autonomous) in which learning algorithms are self-correcting. The process by which this self-
correction takes place is known as backpropagation. Backpropagation is a recursive process in which output data
can be recycled through the layers of the deep neural network and the weight of each connection is readjusted to
reduce errors. With each iteration, the accuracy of the
probability calculated increases.

Though Hinton had published his groundbreaking
paper on a learning algorithm for backpropagation in 1986,
he did not make his final mathematical breakthrough until
2005. In a 2019 interview, he recalls this critical turning
point. In response to a question about whether he ever
doubted that neural networks were viable, Hinton explains,
"Something like this has to work. I mean, the connections
in the brain are learning somehow, and we just have to figure it out. And probably there's a bunch of different ways
of learning connection strengths; the brain's using one of
them. There may be other ways of doing it. But certainly you
have to have something that can learn these connection
strengths. I never doubted that." He then proceeds to
recount how he arrived at his most important insight while
working on the analysis of images.

> In about 2005, I came up with a way of doing unsuper-
> vised training of deep nets. So you take your input, say
> your pixels, and you'd learn a bunch of feature detectors
> that were just good at explaining why the pixels were even
> like that. And then you treat those feature detectors as the
> data, and you learn another bunch of feature detectors, so
> we could explain why those feature detectors have those

correlations. And you keep learning layers and layers. But what was interesting was, you could do some math and prove that each time you learned another layer, you didn't necessarily have a better model of the data, but you had a band on how good your model was. And you could get a better band each time you added another layer.[21]

Suppose you wanted to train a machine to recognize a picture of a horse. If you were using symbolic AI, it would be necessary first to provide a program with a precise definition or description of a horse and then supply the machine with instructions to identify the images as horse or not-horse. In practice, it is almost impossible to give a definition that will allow the computer to avoid errors. Deep learning in neural networks proceeds in the opposite direction by moving from images to concept rather than from concept to image. In neither supervised (semiautonomous) nor unsupervised (autonomous) neural networks is the machine given a definition or a description of a horse or the rules for identifying a horse. In supervised neural network learning, the input is structured data labeled horse/not-horse. After processing a sufficient number of images, the networks learn how to distinguish horse from not-horse in images that have not been tagged. In unsupervised neural networks, the desired output is specified, but input data are not labeled or structured. The network is fed random images, only some of which are of horses, and through a process of trial and error the network identifies some images as horse. This success is reinforced by adjusting the weights of the relevant inputs, and errors are corrected through the process of backpropagation. This procedure requires no human intervention after it has started. The initial results of unsupervised learning were disappointing. It turned out that the problem was scale—there were not enough images for neural networks to practice on. In recent years, this situation has changed dramatically with images from the Internet, YouTube, Instagram, Facebook, and many other online media. The convergence of all of these factors has led to the current AI revolution.

It is important to understand that neural networks produce probabilities rather than certainties. In other words, deep learning cannot identify the image of a horse with 100 percent certainty, but can only determine the range of probability that any given image is a horse. The emphasis on probability and not certainty was one of the primary factors that made so many computer scientists suspicious of neural networks for so long. The second point to underscore is that the structure and operational procedures of neural networks can be used to analyze all kinds of data. What makes neural networks unique is that the algorithm for computing the function is not produced by encoding a proven formula or procedure for computing the output, but rather by adjusting the parameters to a simple general-purpose computational model based solely on having access to multiple inputs and outputs derived from the data. Neural networks and the deep learning they enable make the Internet of Things and the Internet of Bodies possible.

To understand how neural networks and deep learning operate in the real world, it is helpful to return to the games of chess and Go. While Deep Blue used symbolic AI to defeat Kasparov, the greater complexity of Go made this approach untenable. Using the advances in neural networks, a group of young computer scientists who had studied at Cambridge University developed an alternative to IBM's strategy. To test the theory, they proposed to create a machine that could defeat the world's greatest Go player. In 2010, Demis Hassabis, Mustafa Suleyman, and Shane Legg founded the London-based company Deep-Mind to explore the possibility of using neural networks to create new types of AI that could advance research in different areas and to solve the most difficult real-world problems. To accomplish this lofty ambition, they started with seemingly inconsequential games. On the company website, they explain, "By implementing our research in the field of games, a useful training ground, we were able to create *a single program* that taught itself how to play and win at 49 completely different Atari titles, with just raw pixels as input. And in a global first, our AlphaGo program took on the world's best player at Go—one of the most complex and intuitive games ever devised, with more positions than there are atoms in the universe—and won."[22] Even the simplest iteration of the network surprised its creators by developing unexpected tactics to win games. In a paper on their early efforts published in *Nature* (2015), the DeepMind team reported, "We demonstrate that the deep Q-network agent, receiving only the pixels and game score inputs, was able to surpass the performance of all previous algorithms and achieve a level comparable to that of a professional human games tester across a set of 49 games."[23]

In 2014, Google acquired DeepMind, which they hoped would create internal competition with their initial AI research project Google Brain. Within a year, engineers at DeepMind had developed AlphaGo and challenged Fan

Hui, who was the reigning European champion at the time, to a five-game match. In preparation for the match, AlphaGo first played 100,000 games of Go, which were on the Internet, and then over the course of several months played 30 million games against itself. The result was that AlphaGo defeated Fan Hui 5–0. This was the first time a machine had beaten a human playing Go. But the DeepMind team was not satisfied with this victory—they wanted to defeat the best Go player in the world just as IBM wanted to beat the best chess player in the world. To achieve this goal, the engineers upgraded AlphaGo to AlphaGo Zero. In contrast to AlphaGo, which began its training by replaying games people had played, AlphaGo Zero did not use any data from human games but played millions of games against itself. The word *Zero* was added to underscore the fact that the neural network trained itself without any human assistance. The designers explain, "We subsequently applied our reinforcement learning pipeline to a second instance of AlphaGo Zero using a larger network and over a longer duration. Training again started from completely random behavior and continued for approximately 40 days. Over the course of training, 29 million games of self-play were generated. Parameters were updated from 3.1 million mini-batches of 2,048 positions each."[24] Their efforts culminated in the Google DeepMind Challenge, which took place March 9–15, 2016, in Seoul, South Korea. DeepMind's opponent was Lee Sedol, who was to Go what Kasparov was to chess—he had won eighteen world championship Go matches and was widely regarded as unbeatable.

An excellent documentary film, *Alpha Go*, conveys the extraordinary media hype surrounding the match. While the event passed unnoticed in the United States, it was closely followed by millions of people in South Korea, China, and Japan. Hundreds of members of the press crowded the hotel where the match was held and attended the press conference following each game. The games were even telecast on huge screens on buildings throughout Seoul. At the outset, it was clear that neither Sedol nor the expert commentators knew what the champion was up against. Sedol confidently predicted that he would easily beat AlphaGo Zero 5–0; his confidence was, however, quickly shattered.

Spectators were intrigued by this unknown challenger but had no understanding of what the machine was or how it worked. Before the match started, one of the members of the team patiently explained that AlphaGo Zero has three basic components.

1. A policy network playing by itself millions of high-level games.
2. A value network evaluates board positions and determines the probability of winning for each one.
3. A tree search looks at different variations of the game and calculates alternative future outcomes. AlphaGo Zero looks ahead fifty to sixty moves.

What makes deep learning so valuable is not only the analytic capability of neural networks but also its ability to make predictions about the consequences of different decisions and actions. AlphaGo Zero is designed to identify the move with the highest probability of leading to victory.

Shortly after game 1 began, Sedol's calm confident demeanor gave way to anxious fidgeting. Like Kasparov, Sedol admitted that he had been unnerved by a machine that played like a human being yet showed no emotion and gave no clues about its psychological state. It did not take long for AlphaGo Zero to win the first game. In the press conference following the game, the mood changed—it was clear that for Sedol, as well as the millions of people following the match, the stakes were high. Go was more than a game for them, it was an art that expressed a philosophy of life and revealed the innermost essence of the player. This match involved nothing less than a contest for the future of humanity.

Game 2 was the turning point in the match. When AlphaGo Zero made its thirty-seventh move, there was an audible gasp in the audience, and a baffled look slowly crept across Sedol's face. Puzzled commentators were confident that the machine had made a mistake that created an opening for Sedol. It gradually became apparent, however, that AlphaGo Zero had not made a mistake, but was thinking far ahead and had made a completely original move that no human being ever would have conceived. Though Sedol realized what had occurred and suspected defeat was inevitable, he played on, resisting resigning until he had no other choice. After the game, he reflected on what had happened. "I thought AlphaGo Zero was based on probability and calculation, and I thought it was merely a machine. But when I saw this move, I changed my mind. Surely, AlphaGo Zero is creative. The move was really creative and beautiful. This made me think about Go in a new light. What does creativity mean and what does Go mean? It was really a meaningful move."[25] Once again the mood of the press conference shifted—anxiety about the match gave way to a grim melancholy that reflected the awareness that something fundamental about the future of humanity had changed with that single move.

Game 4 provided some relief. When AlphaGo Zero played in a way even DeepMind engineers could not understand, Sedol won. People responded with ecstatic relief and ran into the street to celebrate the victory of man over machine. Realizing what was happening, Sedol's response was muted. "People felt weak and fragile and this victory showed that we can still hold our own. In the future it will be very hard to play AlphaGo Zero but winning this one time felt like enough. One time was enough." The respite was brief—AlphaGo Zero won game 5, taking the match 4–1.

Sometimes events that change the world pass virtually unnoticed and can only be recognized in retrospect. It is not too much to say that with move 37 in game 2, the axis of the world shifted. Turing insisted that even the most robust AI could not do anything that was new or original and thus could approximate human intelligence but not equal its creativity. AlphaGo Zero proved him wrong by doing something no human being could have imagined. DeepMind engineers conclude their paper on AlphaGo Zero, in which they recount the results of their work, with a startling claim.

Our results comprehensively demonstrate that a pure reinforcement learning approach is fully feasible, even in the most challenging of domains: it is possible to train to a superhuman level, without human examples for guidance, given no knowledge of the domain beyond basic rules. Furthermore, a pure reinforcement approach requires just a few more hours to train, and achieves much better asymptotic performance, compared to training on human expert data. Using this approach, AlphaGo Zero defeated the strongest previous versions of AlphaGo, which were trained from human data using handcrafted features, by a large margin.

Humankind has accumulated Go knowledge from millions of games played over thousands of years, collectively distilled into patterns, proverbs and books. In the space of a few days, starting from *tabula rasa*, AlphaGo Zero was able to rediscover much of this Go knowledge, as well as novel strategies that provide new insights into the oldest of games.[26]

As we will see in chapter 5, the emergence of superintelligence marks a new stage in evolution that simultaneously includes and surpasses human being as we have known it.

Not everyone missed the importance of AlphaGo Zero's victory. Kai-Fu Lee had worked for Apple, Silicon Graphics, and Microsoft, where he was vice president of Interactive Services. In 2005, he left Microsoft to become the head of Google China and by 2016 he had become a venture capitalist working in Beijing's Zhongguancun, which is China's Silicon Valley. Reflecting on the victory of AI over human intelligence, he writes, "To people here, AlphaGo's victories were both a challenge and an inspiration. They turned into China's 'Sputnik Moment' for artificial intelligence."[27] When

Lee looks to the future, he sees an emerging world order created by a new cold war between the United States and China for dominance in artificial intelligence.

One of the reasons so many people have missed the significance of AlphaGo Zero is that they have misunderstood what artificial intelligence is and how it works. When AI is mentioned, there is a tendency for people to think about films like *The Terminator* and *Star Wars's* R2-D2, or humanoid robots. While some researchers are exploring whole brain emulation, which simulates human intelligence, currently more important forms of AI are being used for information processing and quasi-cognitive tasks that require neither consciousness nor self-consciousness. As the mission statement of DeepMind suggests, these emerging technologies have a remarkably broad range of applications.

> We're on a scientific mission to push the boundaries of AI, developing programs that can learn to solve any complex problem without needing to be taught how. If we're successful, we believe this will be one of the most important and widely beneficial scientific advances ever made, increasing our capacity to understand the mysteries of the universe and to tackle some of the most pressing real-world challenges. From climate change to the need for radically improved healthcare, too many people suffer from painfully slow progress, their complexity overwhelming our ability to find solutions. With AI as a multiplier for human ingenuity, those solutions will come into reach.[28]

Inevitably, however, commercial interests take over technological innovations and use them for financial gain. Just as the Internet was created to facilitate communication among university researchers and then was commercialized, so new forms of AI developed to solve urgent environmental and social problems have been appropriated to create a relentless money machine that has led to the greatest disproportion of wealth in history. This situation shows no signs of changing—to the contrary, the very structure and operation of complex positive feedback networks create accelerating returns that will lead to increasing disparities.

A recent report from the World Economic Forum entitled "Personal Data: The Emergence of a New Asset Class" suggests where all of this is heading.

We are moving towards a "Web of the world" in which mobile communications, social technologies, and sensors are connecting people, the Internet and the physical world into one interconnected network. Data records are collected on who we are, who we know, where we are, where we have been and where we plan to go. Mining and analyzing this data give us the ability to understand and even predict where humans focus their attention and activity at the individual, group, and global level. . . . At its core, personal data represents a post-industrial opportunity. It has unprecedented complexity, velocity and global reach. Utilizing a ubiquitous communications infrastructure, personal data will emerge in a world where nearly everyone and everything are connected in real time. . . . Stakeholders will need to embrace the uncertainty, ambiguity, and risk of an emerging ecosystem. In many ways this opportunity will resemble a living entity and will require new ways of adapting and responding. Most importantly, it will demand a new way of thinking about individuals.[29]

To understand how fast *things* are changing, it is important to recall how recently the companies deploying these new technologies were created. Amazon was founded in 1994, Google in 1998, and Facebook in 2004. The iPhone was introduced in 2007, and autonomous machine learning was successfully demonstrated in 2016. When Google was created only 7 percent of the population in the United States was connected to the Internet. Since the Internet had been developed by nonprofit institutions, people initially were reluctant to pay for commercial online services, and companies struggled to find ways to make a profit. Almost all early business models were based on projected ad revenues calculated by the number of page hits on websites. This strategy proved ineffective because it was impossible to predict who would click on ads. Around 2002, Google executives realized that their search engine was generating an even more lucrative revenue stream by indirectly providing what Shoshana Zuboff describes as a "behavioral surplus." The advent of Big Data has made it possible to use machine learning to develop very valuable predictive analytics. As networks expanded and the number of computer-mediated transactions increased, the amount of data accumulated and stored has grown exponentially. Zuboff quotes Google's chief economist Hal Varian's explanation of the importance of this discovery. " 'Nowadays there is a computer in the middle of virtually every transaction . . . now that they are available these computers have several uses.' He then identifies four such new uses: 'data extraction and analysis,' 'new contractual forms due to better monitoring,' 'personalization and customization,' and 'continuous experiments.' "[30] By using neural networks and machine deep learning to analyze people's search histories, Google can determine the probability an individual will click on an ad and even project the likelihood he or she will purchase the product. In 2003, Google engineers filed a patent for "Generating User Information for Use in Target Advertising." This development marked nothing less than the beginning of a new world that quickly spread to encompass all aspects of life.

As more companies and investors recognized the economic value of the data generated by behavioral surplus, the quest for data expanded from Internet searches and web browsing to mobile phones, Global Position Systems, and preferences for magazines, books, films, music, restaurants, and anything else that provides clues to predict behavior patterns. All of these data are processed by neural networks like those used in AlphaGo. While computer scientists and software engineers were revolutionizing AI, other researchers were developing entirely new digital sensors small enough to embed in almost anything, enabling devices to communicate with computers or mobile phones. "Today's microelectronic technology," Samuel Greengard explains, "measures many more things—and measures them far more accurately—than even the most sophisticated analog and mechanical devices of the past. They can incorporate multiple functions on a single microchip and they rely on a common binary code to transmit and receive data in real time. What's more, connecting a vast array of sensors or building them into machines including robotic devices, provides deep insights into the interrelationships of different factors and systems in the physical world. Simply put, the technology takes us where no man or woman has ever gone before."[31]

These devices can be placed in cars, planes, roads, bridges, and are used extensively in machines, stores, and factories. Some individual oil drilling platforms, for example, have as many as 30,000 embedded sensors. The average car currently has 60–100 sensors, and in the next few years this number is predicted to increase to 200, which translates into 200 billion sensors per year just for the automobile industry. The spread of miniature sensors creates the conditions for pervasive panopticism. Increasingly, sensors are watching us everywhere we go and are recording everything we say and do. Even when you are sleeping, sensors in your iPhone, mattress, clock, and television are collecting and transmitting data. To make matters worse—or better, depending on your point of view—the insatiable demand for data has led to the creation of countless consumer products designed to collect, process, and transmit data. Everything from eyeglasses and toothbrushes to clothes, refrigerators, and shopping carts have or soon will have sensors. According to Greengard, "Cisco Systems estimates that approximately 12.1 billion Internet connected devices were in use in April 2014, and the figure is expected to zoom to above 50 billion by 2020. In fact the networking firm says that about 100 'things' currently connect to the Internet every second but the number will reach 250 per second by 2020. Overall, the Internet Solutions Group at Cisco Systems estimates that more than 1.5 trillion 'things' exist in the physical world and 99 per cent of physical things will eventually become part of the network."[32] Devices with sensors create revenue streams both from the sale of the products and from the sale of the data they generate.

As sensors become smaller and more sophisticated, the range of their applications expands to include all the senses—things not only become smart, they can also see, hear, smell, taste, and touch. With the creation of voice recognition programs, digital assistants, and smart home devices like Siri, Google Assistant, Amazon's Alexa and Echo, things are no longer dumb, and it is possible to have a seemingly meaningful conversation with them. By providing more data to be analyzed and processed by neural networks, deep learning makes these devices increasingly intelligent. The Internet of Things has been created to make these devices even smarter by connecting them to each other. Just as stand-alone computer work stations and personal computers were connected first in local, then wider, and finally global networks, so individual stand-alone devices eventually were connected in networks that operate on algorithms enabling them to communicate with each other.

In many cases, the complexity and speed of the networks make it impossible for human beings to intervene in their operation. Engineers have even produced algorithms that are able to generate other algorithms the smartest computer scientists could never create. These algorithms can process data on the fly from all the devices in a network through super-high-speed feedback loops, creating autonomous machines that continue to learn at a rate far too fast for human beings to keep up with. The result is a real-time constantly intervolving network run by algorithms, with little

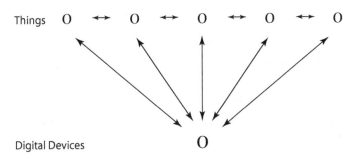

FIGURE 3.3 Internet of Things. Mark C. Taylor.

or no human intervention, that enables connected devices to make constant adjustments to each other through the give-and-take of ever expanding shared data.

By uniting the virtual and the real worlds, the coadaptive Internet of Things lends agency to distributed objects. Shared code and algorithms create communications channels that enable the network to operate as an integrated whole. Because these networks are self-regulating and self-educating, the more they operate, the smarter they become, and the smarter they become, the more they operate. A 2010 report entitled *The Internet of Things* issued by the global consulting firm McKinsey & Co. summarized the significance of these developments. "The predictable pathways of information are changing: the physical world itself is becoming a type of information system. . . . These networks churn out huge volumes of data that flow to computers for analysis. When objects can both sense the environment and communicate, they become tools for understanding complexity and responding to it swiftly. What's revolutionary in all of this is that these physical information systems are now being deployed, and some of them even work largely without human intervention."[33]

The combination of neural networks, deep learning, and the IoT forms the technological unconscious that makes possible many of today's most disruptive innovations. Everything from self-driving cars and self-piloted planes to smart agriculture and smart factories depends on wired networks with smart machines that talk to each other. On a six-hundred-acre strawberry farm in Florida, for example, every single plant has a sensor that monitors it and sends information enabling machines to calculate the precise amount of water and fertilizer each plant needs. Sensors communicate when berries are ready to pick, and algorithms direct robots to distinguish ripe from nonripe berries. For manufacturers obsessed with cost and efficiency, the IoT promises the realization of Frederick Winslow Taylor's dream. Networked smart things and programmed robots eliminate the need for human workers on the factory floor. When a product is finished, robots store it in a warehouse where it remains until an order for it is received. Machines then package, address, and ship the item, and drones or robots transported in self-driving cars deliver it to the consumer's door.

Where Jeff Bezos sees the opportunity for more efficiency and greater profits, others see danger. Kai-Fu Lee warns, "Human civilization has in the past absorbed similar technology-driven shocks to the economy, turning hundreds of millions of farmers into factory workers over the nineteenth and twentieth centuries. But none of these changes ever arrived as quickly as AI. Based on the current trends in technology advancement and adoption, I predict that within fifteen years, artificial intelligence will technically be able to replace around 40 to 50 per cent of jobs in the United States."[34] Reeducating people for high-tech careers will not solve the problem because the disruption of manufacturing and blue-collar jobs is rapidly spreading to white-collar work. AI systems already position baseball players, advise social workers, recommend sentences to judges, tutor anxious students, and advise banks on the reliability of borrowers seeking mortgages. And this is only the beginning.

What is emerging through the Internet of Things is a world of *ambient intelligence* created by smart devices equipped with sensors and transmitters to send data to each other and to users whether or not they want it. This environment is thoroughly interactive—machines influence people, and people consciously and unconsciously influence machines. In these networks, intelligence is no longer limited to brains and minds, or even to computational machines, but is rather distributed in smart things. In this way, our everyday world is always becoming more intelligent and is increasingly capable of quasi-cognitive processes. This is creating an environment of *ubiquitous computing.*

The idea of ubiquitous computing was first introduced in 1991 by Mark Weiser, who was then the head of the Computer Science Laboratory at the Xerox Palo Alto Research Center. He begins his extraordinarily prescient article "The Computer for the Twenty-first Century" by claiming that "the most profound technologies are those that disappear. They weave themselves into the fabric of everyday life until they are indistinguishable from it." He proceeds to predict how cheap, low-power computers with convenient display and software applications will all be connected in networks that render smart devices interoperable.[35] To illustrate his point, Weiser describes a smart home like those that are being widely developed today. Zuboff points out that as early as 2000 an interdisciplinary team at Georgia Tech began the Aware Home experiment, which projected a " 'human-home symbiosis' in which many animate and inanimate processes would be captured by an elaborate network of 'context aware sensors' embedded in the house and by wearable computers worn by the home's occupants. The design called for an 'automated wireless collaboration' between the platform that hosted personal information from the occupants' wearables and a second one that hosted environmental information from the sensors."[36]

Computational environments are no longer theoretical constructs or novel experiments, but are evolving all around us. Whenever your mobile phone has its GPS turned on, embedded sensors are monitoring your movements and transmitting information to computers that know the patterns of your behavior as well as your likes and dislikes. This data is processed in relation to your current location and situation, and recommendations for purchases and activities are sent to your phone. Some stores even have sensors on shelves that can track eye movement. When a person's eye stops briefly on a product, the sensor detects the pause and sends the information to a neural network computer, which processes the data in relation to the person's previous patterns of behavior and calculates the probability of a purchase. To nudge the consumer, coupons for the item can be sent to his or her mobile phone. All this occurs in a matter of seconds. In the near future, smart refrigerators stocked with products bearing embedded sensors will automatically transmit data to smart shopping carts at supermarkets. Upon arrival at the store, the cart will greet the customer personally and display a list of items he or she needs as well as suggest other items again based on past purchasing patterns. This is one of the most extreme forms of targeted marketing that currently is encountered every time a person turns on his or her computer or mobile phone.

As we have seen, motivation for the rapid development of neural networks, deep learning, new AI, and sensors has been largely economic. Capitalism's unsustainable commitment to endless market expansion encourages those who own the data to find new ways to use it to get people to buy stuff they do not need. What makes new AI so attractive to the business world is that predicting probabilities makes it possible to modify human behavior. Real-time processing of Big Data enables machines to program not only other things but also the minds and bodies of individuals. While promoters of the information and AI revolution like Steve Jobs, Tim Cook, Bill Gates, Jeff Bezos, and Mark Zuckerberg preach the gospel of infinite choice, their real goal is to take decisions away from individuals by programming them to want what they want them to want. What Zuboff aptly labels "the commodification of behavior" leads to programmatic behavior modification. Ubiquitous computing creates surveillance networks that are the technological foundation for political and economic systems ranging from surveillance capitalism to rapidly proliferating authoritarian regimes. Zuboff concludes, "An appreciation of the surveillance logic of accumulation that drives this action suggests that this network of things is already evolving into a network of coercion, in which mundane functions are ransomed for behavioral surplus." She quotes a senior software engineer involved with creating the IoT who freely admits that "the real aim is ubiquitous intervention, action, and control. The real power is that now you can *modify* real-time actions in the real world. Connected smart sensors can register and analyze any kind of behavior and then actually figure out how to change it. Real-time analytics translate into real-time action."[37]

106   Increased convenience has a price; the first and most obvious cost is the loss of privacy. Not only are machines constantly watching us and collecting information about us, but we do not even know where our data is, who owns it, or what they are doing with it. This creates an asymmetrical relationship in which we are subjected to the constant gaze of an omniscient other we can never see. Second, the very technologies that create the possibility of mass customization and personalization also negate individuality by programming our minds and bodies. The machines we have programmed to program themselves end up programming us. In this way, we become extensions of and subject to the machines we have created. This is the same dynamic that Hegel saw in the master-slave relationship and Ludwig Feuerbach saw in the man-god relationship.

The potential abuse of the Internet of Things has led many critics to argue that research, development, and deployment of these technologies should be strictly regulated or even terminated.[38] While prudent oversight is undeniably advisable and necessary, it would be a serious mistake to curtail the development of technologies that hold enormous promise for improving our lives and alleviating suffering. The same technologies that are being used by unscrupulous companies for targeted marketing, and by nefarious politicians to control individuals, can also be used by scientists and physicians for vital medical research and the treatment of devastating diseases. In a richly suggestive paper, "Our Extended Sensoria: How Humans Will Connect with the Internet of Things," Joseph Paradiso, who is the director of the MIT Media Lab's Responsive Environment Group, writes,

> We are entering a world where ubiquitous sensor information from our proximity will propagate up into various levels of what is now termed the "cloud" then project back down into our physical and logical vicinity as context to guide processes and applications manifesting around us. . . . Right now, all information is available on many devices around me at the touch of a finger or the enunciation of a phrase. Soon it will stream directly into our eyes and ears once we enter the age of wearables. . . . This information will be driven by context and attention, not direct query, and much of it will be pre-cognitive, happening before we formulate direct questions. Indeed, the boundaries of the individual will be very blurry in this future. . . . In the future, where we will live and learn in a world deeply networked by wearables and eventually

implantables, how our essence and individuality is bro-
kered between organic neurons and whatever the information ecosystem becomes is a fascinating frontier that
promises to redefine humanity.[39]

The frontier where the Internet of Things meets the Internet of Bodies is the digital pancreas I wear on my belt.

4

Internet of Bodies

Where does my body begin? Where does it end? What is inside my body? What is outside? What is primary? What is secondary? What is natural? What is artificial? What is original? What is supplemental? In his exceptionally illuminating book, *Prosthesis*, literary critic David Wills writes,

> Where would such a thing, a prosthesis, have to start in order to have started? How would it begin? To be made, built, or constructed? To be told or written? . . . Any occlusion at the beginning is the effect of transfer, the fact of its being already in process. . . . From earthbound gallop to quadrupedantic flight, from leg of flesh to leg of steel, it is necessary to transfer otherness, articulated through the radical alterity of ablation as loss of integrity. And this otherness is mediated through the body, works through the operation of a transitive verb . . . signifying first of all something carried by the body. In translation, what is

carried across or transferred is borne by the body. But it doesn't just carry itself; it carries a self that is divided in its function—walking, carrying. Before it begins to carry anything external to itself it bears that effect of its own internal scission. Thus it is the otherness that the body must carry in order to move that begins—and a first-person adjective is now ready to bear it—this is our prosthesis.[1]

Our bodies. Our selves. A body divided, a self split, an I doubled. Not just my body, my self, my I, but everyone's. This is the otherness that I, that we must bear not only to move but also to be.

Writers and artists often glimpse the future before the scientists and engineers who create it. Few people have been more willing to put their bodies on the line for the future they envision than the Cyprus-born performance artist Stelarc. Throughout his career, Stelarc has been preoccupied with the bodily effects of information technologies. To explore the implications of changes now occurring, he has transformed his body into a constantly morphing work of art by swallowing miniature cameras, then projecting their movement through his intestines, and by adding prostheses like a robotic third arm activated by electromyography (EMG) signals transmitted from his abdominal muscles. In another experiment, he grafted a biologically engineered third ear onto his arm. Geeta Dayal reports her interview with Stelarc: "'At present it's only a relief of an ear,' Stelarc said. 'When the ear becomes a more 3-D structure we'll reinsert the small microphone that connects a wireless transmitter.' In any Wi-Fi hotspot, he said, it will become

Internet-enabled. 'So if you're in San Francisco and I'm in London, you'll be able to listen in to what my ear is hearing, wherever you are and wherever I am.'"[2] In one of his most prescient works, Stelarc literally makes himself a prosthesis of a prosthesis by wiring himself to machines that viewers can use to activate his body remotely.

In 1995, he staged "Ping Body" in Paris, Helsinki, and Amsterdam. During the performance, his body was not moved by his own nervous system but by the flow of data on the Internet. Stelarc explains the performance.

> By random pinging (or measuring the echo times) to Internet domains it is possible to map spatial distance and transmission time to body motion. Ping values from

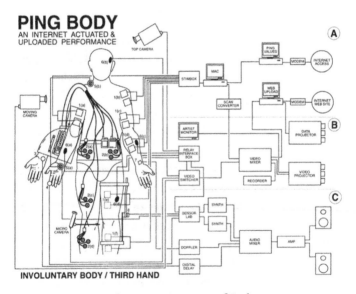

FIGURE 4.1 Ping Body. Image courtesy of Stelarc.

0–2000 milliseconds (indicative of both distance and density levels of Internet activity) are used to activate a multiple muscle stimulator directing 0–60 volts to the body. Thus ping values that indicate spatial and time parameters of the Internet choreograph and compose the performances. A graphical interface of limb motions simulates and initiates the physical body's movements. This, in turn, generates sounds mapped to proximity, positioning and bending of the arms and legs. The Ping Body performances produce a powerful inversion of the usual interface of the body to the Net. Instead of collective bodies determining the operation of the Internet, collective Internet activity moves the body. The Internet becomes not merely a mode of information transmission, but also a transducer, effecting physical action.[3]

While the Internet of Things creates distributed cognition by connecting smart devices, Stelarc's performative experiments point toward an Internet of Bodies that creates smart interactive distributed bodies.

Our investigation of disease has shown the inadequacy of the long-standing tradition that establishes an opposition between mind and body. The body, we discovered, is an information-processing network whose structure and operation mirror neural networks in the brain. More precisely, the investigation of the intricacies of the immune system reveals the body to be a network of interactive networks that form a bodily Intranet, which does not form a completely closed loop. When the immune system turns against itself in autoimmune diseases, it exposes an other within the body that creates the opening for connecting the Intranet of the Body to the Internet of Things and the Internet of other bodies. The IoT consists of separate as well as networked devices that can be either prostheses or implants in the human body.

The proliferation of neural networks and deep learning has led to the invention of much more sophisticated implants than Stelarc envisioned. Updating Stelarc's internal body camera, engineers are now developing the hardware and software for a camera that can be used to perform a virtual colonoscopy. Patients swallow a camera that projects a 3-D video that is analyzed by algorithms to detect cancerous or precancerous polyps with a high degree of accuracy. Devices that can be swallowed are not limited to cameras—there is also a whole new generation of pills that is being used for diagnostic and treatment purposes. Scientists at Australia's Royal Melbourne Institute of Technology have created a pill that measures gases in the intestine as food passes through it. By detecting traces of oxygen, hydrogen, and carbon dioxide, doctors can diagnose digestive disorders. Some pills are even capable of administering injections while they are in the digestive tract. The capsules have tiny needles filled with drugs that can puncture the intestine wall and release medication. Researchers are exploring whether these devices can be used to administer insulin for diabetics. MIT scientists have created an ingestible Origami Robot that has computation capability embedded in it. The device, which is made of biodegradable material, is equipped with magnets and sensors and can be controlled from outside the body. So far the robot has been used to remove foreign objects and repair wounds in an artificial stomach. Eventually, scientists expect it to be able to deliver medications and even perform surgeries.

Recent advances in nanotechnology have carried miniaturization all the way down to the molecular level. This breakthrough has created new applications for the bodily deployment of artificial intelligence. In an informative article entitled "Robotics and the Internet of Bodies," Ernesto Rodriguez Leal, who is professor of robotics at the Monterrey Institute of Technology, anticipates a broad range of developments in the near future.

> With such IoT devices—and the embedded sensors they contain—it is now possible to track biometric data such as heart rate, oxygen levels in the blood, and physical activity non-invasively. Add to this recent developments in skin electronics, harvesting energy from body thermodynamics, and new biocompatible materials. In the future we'll see implantable devices that will lead us toward a set of Internet of Body technologies.
>
> We can expect to use nanobots that flow through our body, able to transmit information such as body temperature, blood chemistry, biomarkers, insulin levels, arterial pressure, and flow wirelessly. And this will be interpreted by AI-based algorithms, which will in turn use all of this data and its correlations to warn of possible diseases early on. These nanobots will also have other functions: mimicking white blood cells to protect the body from diseases or performing swarm collaboration to intervene in case of trauma to regenerate the body.[4]

As internal and external prostheses become more sophisticated, the range of their functionality expands. ABILIFY MYCITE has developed a system to monitor medication.

A patient swallows a pill with a sensor and wears a patch that records the date and time medication was taken as well as the person's level of activity. The patch communicates this information to an app on the patient's smartphone, and a web-based portal gives healthcare providers access to the information and the ability to communicate with the patient about adjustments in dosage. Countless such devices are being developed to monitor patients' activities and intervene when necessary. The advent of 3-D printing makes it possible to use these data to produce customized prostheses and devices.

These technological innovations are transforming the very structure and operation of minds and bodies as well as changing the way they interact. While these devices are connected to and communicate with networks of the patient's healthcare providers, they are not yet connected with other devices the patient is using or the devices and networks of other patients, physicians, or data managers. Just as connecting stand-alone computers in local and eventually global networks represented a quantum leap in computational capacity, and wiring individual things in an IoT greatly enhanced the power of individual devices, so the wiring of bodies first to the IoT and then to other bodies is not only transforming healthcare but also redefining human subjects. As the Intranet of the Body is connected to the Internet of Bodies through the Internet of Things, individual bodies as well as the networks connecting them learn faster and become smarter. These developments create irresistible opportunities for leading high-tech companies. Using the same technologies that enabled them to disrupt manufacturing, communications, media, commerce, and finance, these companies are now developing strategies to disrupt healthcare.

With an aging population and an increasing number of people suffering from costly chronic diseases like diabetes, the $3.5 trillion healthcare industry in the United States is ripe for change. Waste and inefficiency could be significantly reduced by using artificial intelligence to perform many of the same tasks being done less adequately by human beings. Google, Amazon, and IBM, as well as many smaller and less powerful companies are partnering with leading hospitals and clinics to change every aspect of healthcare. In the process, they are literally reengineering the body in ways that will lead to a new stage in evolution.

The consulting firm CBINSIGHTS uses AI to advise their clients on companies and innovations that have the greatest probability of yielding high returns on investments. Not surprisingly, many of the companies they recommend are using the same technologies in their own businesses. Their report entitled "How Google Plans to Use AI to Reinvent the $3 Trillion US Healthcare Industry" begins:

> Google is betting that the future of healthcare is going to be structured data and AI. The company is applying AI to disease detection, new data infrastructure, and potentially insurance. . . .
>
> Google has always seen itself as more than a search and advertising company.
>
> Now it's turning its focus to healthcare, betting that its AI prowess can create a powerful new paradigm for the detection, diagnosis, and treatment of disease.[5]

Google's "AI prowess" is largely the result of their timely acquisition of DeepMind. The hardware and software they are using in their healthcare initiatives are the same they used to beat Lee Sedol in games of Go.

Google's DeepMind is also building a new data infrastructure through its initiatives. DeepMind is looking for ways to apply artificial intelligence and analytics to improve healthcare. To accomplish this, they need access to data in usable, consistently structured formats.

DeepMind's first step is to build a new data infrastructure so that separate, siloed data from EMRs [electronic medical records], hospital equipment, and doctor's notes flow into a singular place in one standard format.

Using FHIR [fast healthcare interoperability resources], DeepMind built a new data backbone to make it easier to build apps that can analyze different data elements.

For example, the company unveiled its "Streams" app to detect acute kidney injuries by pushing relevant patient information and alerts to doctors, nurses, etc. via a mobile app. This reduces the number of humans involved in escalating the severity of a case, which is especially useful when a case is time sensitive.[6]

Though the area of application is different, the technology and business plan are the same as in all other areas Google is taking over.

In addition to supporting research on free-standing and single-loop medical devices, Google, along with other companies, is working to create instruments that can be used in robotic surgery. While surgical robots have been around for more than thirty years, the development of new forms of artificial intelligence has led to dramatic improvements in their performance. Like insulin pumps, new surgical systems can be either semiautonomous or autonomous. Just as machine learning is leading to the disappearance of car and truck drivers and airplane pilots, so too deep learning will lead to a significant reduction in the number of surgeons needed to perform many operations. Echoing Ray Kurzweil in a *Scientific American* article entitled "The Surgical Singularity Is Approaching," Stanford neurosurgeon fellow Sandip Panesar writes,

> In 2016, the Smart Tissue Anastomosis Robot (STAR), an autonomous surgical robot, underwent experimental trials in animals. The robot, which utilized "smart sensing" apparatus including cameras and mechanical sensors, along with AI-control algorithms, outperformed human surgeons at certain tasks, including joining intestines in a living animal without *direct human intervention.* . . . STAR had to perform multiple real-time tasks simultaneously, while minimizing risk of collateral damage: "seeing" the environment in which it was working, "sensing" the features of the tissue upon which it was operating, and "reacting" to environmental changes as they occurred, mimicking human surgeons' "judgment" in addition to their physical skill.[7]

As we have seen, deep learning requires massive amounts of data. For these data to be useful to AI, they must be homogenous and easily searchable. The problem of reaching agreement about data standardization remains unresolved. According to Mark Michalski and Ittai Dayan, codirectors of the data analytics branch of Boston's Partners HealthCare, the chief impediment to improving data analysis, and thus patient outcomes, is not technological but rather the issue of patient privacy. A recent court case shows the reason for their concern. In 2017, Google and the University of Chicago Medical Center formed a partnership to share patient data in electronic medical records for the purposes of analyzing the data using artificial intelligence with the hope of discovering new treatments and possibly cures for a broad range of diseases. According to a *New York Times* report, a class-action lawsuit accuses the university hospital of "sharing hundreds of thousands of patients' records without stripping identifiable date stamps or doctor's notes." Daisuke Wakabayashi explains the far-reaching ramifications of this case. "The suit . . . demonstrates the difficulties technology companies face in handling health data as they forge ahead into one of the most promising—and potentially lucrative—areas of artificial intelligence: diagnosing medical problems. Until policies and procedures for dealing with the privacy matters that are acceptable to all parties are established, medical research will be prevented from taking advantage of one of its most valuable sources of information."[8]

As more data become available to more engineers, companies and healthcare providers, AI will play an increasingly important role in research and clinical applications. Innovation will be most notable in five areas.

Diagnostics
Prediction and prevention

Prescription

Intervention

Patient monitoring and behavior modification

To gain a better understanding of the contributions of AI to establishing an effective Internet of Bodies, it is helpful to consider two areas where the technology is relatively advanced: image analytics and voice recognition.

For the general public, the most widely known application of AI for image analytics is facial recognition. Businesses, governments, militaries, and law enforcement officials are already using facial recognition programs to monitor behavior. The miniaturization of sensors and cameras creates a panoptical environment in which there is a steady flow of images from many places at all times. In addition to this, images from the Internet as well as multiple other media are gathered in data banks for analysis. These images are processed exactly like the horse images I described earlier. In a manner similar to how AlphaGo Zero played millions of games before it could win its match, deep learning networks figure out how to identify the face they are looking for by processing millions of images. This technology is directly transferable to medical applications. So far, the most successful use of image analytics in healthcare is in radiology. In medicine, as in Go, success depends on pattern recognition.

Deep learning programs are now being used to analyze images from X-rays and MRIs. To get a sense of the scope of this technology, consider the fact that for each MRI performed, up to 30,000 images are uploaded to the cloud for visual analysis. By 2015, General Electric had already connected 500,000 MRI machines globally. According to Topol, "All told, there are more than 800 million medical scans a year in the United States, which amounts to about 60 billion images, or one image generated every two seconds." Furthermore, two billion X-rays are done each year worldwide.[9] Since 2012, there has been an explosive growth in the use of machine learning for analyzing medical images. As machines have processed more images, they have gotten smarter and their error rate has plummeted.

One of the most successful applications of deep learning is the analysis of MRIs of tumors. By processing millions of images, neural networks learn how to recognize relevant patterns that indicate the present state of tumors. Machines can do this much faster and for a much lower cost than human radiologists. A 2017 study found a 97 percent accuracy for breast cancer detection, more than 90 percent for esophageal cancer, 95 percent for lung cancer, and 97 percent for diabetic retinopathy. In addition to this, AI is able to personalize or individualize the analysis of tumors. Each person's tumor is unique, and, therefore, not all tumors for a particular disease should be treated the same way. AI is able to "read" the unique fingerprint of a tumor by identifying distinct patterns that are not visible to the human eye. This information can be used to develop a customized treatment for patients. The increased accuracy and efficiency in the use of AI for analyzing images leaves little doubt that within a very short time all medical records will be analyzed and recommendations as well as decisions about treatment made by algorithms running on autonomous neural networks. It is becoming apparent that radiology is a dying specialization for human beings.

Image analytics also have predictive value. In many cases, machine learning can identify latent tumors or signs of a disease up to five years before the human eye can. This capability enables AI to diagnose much earlier than physicians and make recommendations for the best course of treatment by either specifying customized drugs or proposing a customized surgical strategy. For example, predictive algorithms similar to those used in financial markets can be used for risk management in surgery. On the basis of the data analyzed, algorithms can assess the likelihood of a patient developing complications from different surgical procedures and predict how patients are likely to react to different medications. With sufficient data on a person's medical history and patterns of behavior, deep learning can even predict the probability of opioid addiction. While machines do not yet make final decisions about treatment, they increasingly define the parameters within which doctors make their decisions.

When these techniques are combined with recent developments in telecommunications technologies, additional innovations become possible. Telemedicine promises to disrupt medical practice as much as online education and tele-classrooms are disrupting education. Real-time image analysis and semiautonomous or autonomous robotic surgical devices make it possible for surgeons to operate on anyone anywhere in the world at any time. Smart machines extend the eyes and hands of the surgeon around the entire globe. A report recently released by the University of Buffalo's Jacobs Institute predicts that by 2045 the majority of surgical tasks will be performed by robots overseen by humans. "Open platforms allow for plug and play for different functionality (instrumentation, visualization, robot-ics), giving the surgeon unmatched flexibility. Currently, a surgeon is 'locked into' using a particular robot's instru-mentation and visualization and software. In 10 years, a surgeon will be able to choose visualization from one com-pany and instrumentation from another."[10] Interoperability among real-time image processing machines as well as robotic devices eventually will take many human surgeons out of the loop.

As data expand to include more than images, the func-tionality of machine learning becomes even more impress-ive. AI is now being used to assist physicians in making decisions during childbirth. Blood pressure, the heart and respiration rates, and other relevant data on a child's condi-tion are transmitted to a neural network, where they are analyzed using additional personal information stored in electronic medical records to determine how a woman and her child will react to different medications. Again, all of this is done in real time. Like a machine recommending stocks to an investor or player positions to a baseball man-ager, machines calculate probabilities and give physicians alternative options among which they can choose. A more general application of machine learning has even more far-reaching implications for wiring together bodies and machines. In addition to being used for diagnosis, predic-tion, and prescription, AI can also actively intervene in treat-ment procedures. Deep learning machines can analyze an individual's data, determine the specific drug and dose needed, and deliver the medication either with or without human oversight. Automated drug infusion systems are already being used in operating rooms and intensive care units. This innovation can also be used to monitor patients, deliver reminders about taking medicine, or actually administer the medication through implanted or wearable devices.[11] Vinod Khosla, cofounder of Sun Microsystems, goes so far as to claim, "It is inevitable that, in the future, the majority of physicians' diagnosis, prescription, and monitoring, which over time may approach 80 percent of total doctors'/internists' time spent on medicine, will be replaced by smart hardware, software, and testing."[12]

The revival of neural networks has made it possible to develop new uses for natural language processing, which adds additional features to the IoB. Natural language processing has been around since the 1950s, but the dominance of symbolic AI limited its effectiveness. With the growth of neural networks and machine learning, the capabilities of these language-processing programs have improved exponentially. Today natural language processing can be used to analyze written or voice texts as well as to facilitate text-to-text and voice-to-text systems. One of the challenges busy physicians face is keeping up with research developments in their areas of expertise. Over two million peer-reviewed articles are published in medical journals each year. AI is being used to "read" these articles, identify studies relevant to a physician's area of expertise, and summarize the conclusions the investigators reached. Text-to-speech software can translate the results into an audio format. This information can be used to keep physicians informed and, when combined with data gleaned from a patient's electronic medical records and behavioral patterns, can contribute to the finding solutions to an individual's problems.

Voice recognition algorithms are even more disruptive than text-based systems. In an effort to alleviate healthcare providers' workloads, engineers are using AI to develop virtual avatars, which serve as physician's assistants that can perform designated tasks. Even more uncanny, these speaking avatars are designed to collect data by interviewing patients. Topol cites a study that reached a surprising conclusion: in many cases, people prefer talking with virtual assistants than with a real person. In an article entitled "It's Only a Computer: Virtual Humans Increase Willingness to Disclose," Jonathan Gratch reports, "By every measure, participants were willing to disclose much more when they thought they were communicating with a virtual human rather than a real one. A couple of participants who interacted with the virtual human conveyed this very well: 'This is way better than talking to a person. I don't really feel comfortable talking about personal stuff to other people.' And 'A human being would be judgmental. I shared a lot of personal things and it was because of that.'"[13] As in chatrooms and some social media, anonymity and impersonality tend to make people more willing to share intimate details about their lives, so patients tend to be more open with virtual assistants than with actual doctors. When people become more accustomed to talking to Siri and Alexa, they will become even more willing to engage with virtual avatars regarding their medical condition. Deepening these relationships will make avatars smarter and enable them to advise and counsel patients.

Voice recognition applications expand the range of devices from which data can be collected and thus increase the diagnostic efficacy and clinical utility of machine learning. The data AI analyzes are not limited to medical images and records but also include information gathered from mobile phones as well as all kinds of wearable devices. Smart machines can diagnose some diseases and predict imminent medical emergencies like seizures, strokes, and depression by registering changes in patterns of voice modulation and typing rhythms on mobile phones or by detecting changes in facial expressions using image analytics. When impending problems are detected, algorithms either can communicate directly with the person, who can take preventive action, or with healthcare providers who can assist the patient. While smart bombs target enemies, and image analytics target criminals and political dissenters, smart machines target smart medical devices that monitor patients and intervene at critical moments.

To increase the usefulness of smart machines and things, it has been necessary to expand the range of their efficacy from purely conceptual operations to emotions. The predominance of symbolic AI and cognitive science modeled on it encouraged the identification of cognition with rule-based manipulation of abstract symbols. This, in turn, reinforced the ancient opposition between mind and body, which privileged reason at the expense of the senses and emotions. To make matters worse, the opposition between the mental and the material became gendered in a way that consistently identified reason with men and sense and emotions with women. Given this interpretation of reason, it was impossible to imagine that computers could sense, feel, or have emotions. In the past few decades, this subordination of the body to the mind has begun to erode from multiple directions, and, with this development, the challenge has become to design new kinds of computers. Some psychologists, neuroscientists, and engineers now agree intelligence—be it natural or artificial—that ignores or represses the senses and emotions is inevitably distorted because feelings influence all thinking. Antonio Damasio has been one of the leaders in reestablishing the balance between body and mind. In his book, *The Feeling of What Happens: Body and Emotion in the Making of Consciousness*, he writes, "The first basis for the conscious *you* is a *feeling* [emphasis added], which arises in the re-representation of the *nonconscious proto-self in the process of being modified* within an account which establishes the cause of the modification. The first trick of consciousness is the cre-ation of this account, and its first result is the feeling of knowing."[14] The appreciation of the cognitive value of the emotions and the emotive aspects of cognition requires a more inclusive notion of intelligence than traditional AI and cognitive science present.

A shift in the understanding of mental processes grew out of the convergence of advances in neuroscience and a renewed appreciation for neural networks. These develop-ments encouraged the revival of affect theory, which Silvan Tomkins first introduced in his two-volume study *Affect Imagery, Consciousness* (1962). By the 1980s and 1990s, social and political changes beyond classrooms and labo-ratories simultaneously inspired and reflected changes in the interpretation of cognitive processing. Leading femi-nist scholars like Eve Sedgwick, Lauren Berlant, and Sara Ahmed revived affect theory to expose the undeniable ways in which traditional understandings of mind, body, cognition, and intelligence are based on questionable assumptions about gender. The recognition of the role of affects and the emotions in cognitive processes creates the possibility of a much more inclusive and effective Internet of Bodies.

Turing had already proposed supplying computers with senses, but the reigning theory of symbolic AI discouraged any exploration of this path of inquiry. An early sign of change occurred in 1967 when Nobel laureate Herb Simon argued that any adequate theory of thinking had to include the emotions. It took thirty years for this argument to have a significant impact on computer science. In 1997, Rosalind Picard, director of the Affective Computing Research Group at MIT's Media Lab, published her groundbreaking book, *Affective Computing*. If cognition has an emotional dimension and emotions are in part cognitive, then machines that are not affective cannot simulate human cognition. In other words, symbolic AI is misguided, and thus a different line of inquiry must be pursued. Picard begins her analysis by boldly declaring, "This book proposes that we give computers the ability to recognize, express, and in some cases, 'have' emotions. Is this absurd? Computers are supposed to be paradigms of logic, rationality, and predictability. For many thinkers, these paradigms are the very foundations of intelligence, and have been the focus of computer scientists working fervently to build an intelligent machine. After nearly a half century of research, however, computer scientists have not succeeded in constructing a machine that can reason intelligently with people."[15]

To overcome this impasse, Picard proceeds to argue, it is necessary to create smart things and machines that can recognize and express emotions, even if they cannot always experience emotions like people do. Drawing on the work of Damasio and other neurophysiologists, she claims, "now there is a preponderance of evidence that emotion plays a pivotal role in functions considered essential to intelligence. This new understanding about the role of emotion in humans indicates a need to rethink the role of emotion in computing." Picard is careful to specify exactly what kind of machines she has in mind. "Let me remind the reader, when I refer to 'computers' I mean not just a monitor and keyboard with one or more CPU's, but also computational agents such as software assistants and animated interactive creatures, robots, and a host of other forms of computing devices, including 'wearables.' . . . Any computational system in software or hardware, might be given affective abilities."[16]

Picard remains convinced that the invention of new miniature sensors and cameras, combined with deep learning and neural networks, makes it possible to create computational devices that not only replicate but also expand the human sensorium. If image recognition algorithms can see patterns humans cannot see, then there is no reason affective computers cannot sense things humans are unable to sense and detect feelings and emotions of which humans remain unaware. The remarkable range of projects Picard, her colleagues, and students at the Media Lab are doing gives a sense of the direction and importance of their research.

Affective Cognitive Framework for Machine Learning and Decision Making
Automatic Stress Recognition in Real-Life Situations

On-Screen Intervention for Regulated Breathing
Mobile Health Intervention for Addiction and PTSD
Measuring Arousal During Therapy for Children with
    Autism and ADHD
Real-Time Assessment of Suicidal Thought and
    Behavior[17]

These projects require the development of a new generation of what Picard calls "affective wearables," which are devices that extend the bounds of the body, thereby creating the possibility of communication with ambient intelligence embedded in a person's surroundings.

In an effort to convey possible educational and medical applications for affective wearables, Picard offers an illuminating example of the experience of receiving piano lessons from a personal computer tutor.

> Imagine you are seated with your computer tutor, and suppose that it reads not only your gestural input, musical timing and phrasing, but that it can also read your emotional state. In other words, it not only interprets your musical expression, but also your facial expression and perhaps other physical changes corresponding to your emotional feelings—maybe heart rate, breathing, blood-pressure, muscular tightness, and posture. Assume it could have the ability to distinguish the three emotions we all appear to have at birth—distress, interest, and pleasure. Given affect recognition, the computer tutor might gauge if it is maintaining your interest during the lesson, before you quit out of frustration and it is too late to try something different.[18]

What a computer piano tutor can do, a computer physician or physician's assistant can also do. If these devices can be created, affective wearables connected to deep learning machines will be used to monitor all kinds of bodily functions and activities. The devices worn by an individual can be connected with other devices to create a wireless personal area network (PAN), which can communicate with other PANs as well as wider networks in which transmitted data can be processed and the results sent back to modify the device or modify the behavior of the person wearing it.

As word of the work of Picard and her colleagues spread, others began to develop devices and apps designed to facilitate affective computing. Watches, fitbits, skin patches, and even mattresses can record and transmit information about cardiac activity, blood pressure, body fat, temperature, respiration, perspiration, stress, anxiety, sleep patterns, eating habits, and exercise routines. This information is uploaded to the cloud and, after instant processing, provides real-time feedback via smartphone apps. The popular Apple Watch can monitor a remarkable range of biometrics and, when connected to its HealthKit app, can store and quickly access a person's health records, including information about chronic diseases, allergies, medications. In addition to continuously recording vital statistics, the watch can generate an electrocardiogram every thirty seconds by simply touching the wristband. Other researchers are working on more subtle and complex affective devices. Some of the most innovative work is being done by John Roberts at Northwestern University. Roberts explains that his research seeks to understand and exploit interesting characteristics of "soft" materials, such as polymers, liquid crystals, and biological tissues, and hybrid combinations of them with unusual classes of inorganic and micro/nanomaterials—ribbons, wires, membranes, tubes. Our aim is to control and induce novel electronic and photonic responses in these materials and to develop new "soft lithographic" and biomimetic approaches for patterning them and guiding their growth. This work combines fundamental studies with forward-looking engineering efforts in a way that promotes positive feedback between the two. . . . These efforts are highly multidisciplinary, and combine expertise from nearly every traditional field of technical study.[19]

If this line of research turns out to be fruitful, there is no reason wearable devices will be limited to watches, wristbands, belt-worn computers, and clothing fabric; rather, they will actually be integrated with bodily tissues and processes. Needless to say, this would greatly expand the functionality of affective computing.

The integration of smart bodies, smart things, and smart machines through wearable affective computing devices creates new possibilities for interactions in ubiquitous computing environments. Communication of implanted and wearable devices with ambient intelligence surrounding an individual's personal area network creates a network of networks with expanding and changing channels of communication. The technology used in smart houses and smart hospitals and clinics can be adapted to other settings where embedded sensors create surveillance networks that constantly monitor the physical and psychological condition of people. Imagine an elderly person who cannot remember when to take her medicine or a person who is prone to falling. Imagine a person with a chronic heart condition that leaves him susceptible to heart attacks. Imagine a person inclined to addiction who attempts to hide alcohol or drugs, or a brittle diabetic who forgets to take insulin and is always at risk of slipping into a coma. Imagine a child with severe learning disabilities who can't manage for herself or an autistic child subject to outbursts of anger and violent behavior. Imagine a young person who suffers depression and is inclined to suicide. In all these cases, and countless others, smart devices interacting with a ubiquitous computing environment can help to modify behavior and provide an intelligent setting that sustains a productive life. For now, most of the machines and networks used to create these environments are overseen and managed by human beings, but in the near future they will increasingly become autonomous.

With this understanding of smart bodies and smart things, it is time to return to Stelarc's Ping Body and my artificial pancreas. Almost three decades ago, Stelarc foresaw the transformation of things, minds, and bodies that emerging information and telecommunications technologies would bring about. Rather than isolated individuals, we have become *nodular subjects*; that is to say, we are nodes in expansive and invasive networks that connect us with other things, bodies, and minds, which combine to constitute our identities in and through our identification with and difference from others. In Stelarc's visionary work, the body extends beyond its ostensible boundaries and is literally wired to other bodies that are connected in an Internet of

Bodies. Stelarc's body is not merely his own but is also influenced and even activated by the deliberate intervention of remote agents. Moreover, and even more surprising, Stelarc's body is stimulated by signals generated by Internet traffic among anonymous agents in the cloud. After considering these recent technological developments, it is worth quoting Stelarc's conclusion about his Ping Body performance again: "Instead of collective bodies determining the operation of the Internet, collective Internet activity moves the body. The body becomes not merely a mode of information transmission, but also a transducer, effecting physical action."[20]

In his exploration of the networked body, Stelarc did not consider how the body in itself is already a smart information and communications network. Our investigation of the immune system and autoimmune disease has revealed the body to be a complex Intranet in which the self is never simply identical to itself, but is always also at the same time the other of itself. This other, which is an outside that is inside, opens the body to more encompassing networks without which it cannot survive. The Intranet of the Body intersects with the Internet of Things and the Internet of Bodies in the artificial pancreas I wear on my belt.

My artificial pancreas brings together all the technologies and functionalities I have been considering: artificial intelligence, high-speed computers, neural networks, deep machine learning, wireless networks, sensors, transmitters, Big Data, mobile devices, wearable computational machines. While most of these instruments were originally designed for military, law enforcement, and commercial reasons, their most important functions are being adapted for

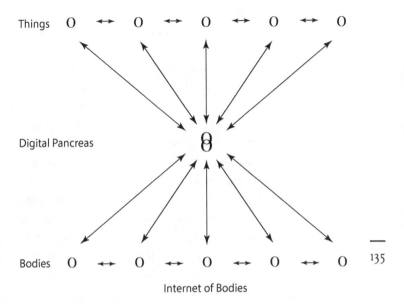

Internet of Bodies

FIGURE 4.2 Intranet of the Body—Internet of Things—Internet of Bodies. Mark C. Taylor.

medical purposes that are increasingly important for the treatment of diseases like diabetes: quantification, personalization, surveillance, communication, ubiquitous computing, ambient intelligence, intervention, and behavior modification.

The transferability of technology from one to another application has encouraged major tech firms like Google and Amazon to expand their market by entering the growing field of healthcare. Both companies recently have undertaken major initiatives in the treatment of diabetes. Google has initiated a series of "moonshot" projects designed to explore the most innovative and risky initiatives. One of the first proposals was a collaboration with Alcon, a global leader in eyecare, to develop a way to measure glucose levels in tears. Other companies are using image analytics to detect diabetic retinopathy. The success rate for this method is 95.9 percent, which is considerably higher than the best trained ophthalmologist. The eye is also an important window to the body that often reveals symptoms of a myriad of diseases. Google's most successful collaboration so far has been its work with Dexcom to create the most effective continuous glucose monitor currently available. An implanted sensor measures glucose levels every five minutes and communicates the information to a transmitter that uses Bluetooth wireless technology to send data to a receiver, mobile phone, or insulin pump. This is the CGM sensor that is embedded in my body.

As I have explained, for type 1 diabetes (that is, insulin-dependent diabetes), there are two types of insulin delivery—basal, which is a more-or-less steady drip, and bolus, which is calculated on the basis of carbohydrate intake and other variables. For people using insulin pumps, the basal rate can be either calculated and set at different fixed rates throughout the day or adjusted automatically by the pump on the basis of glucose monitor readings. In both types of pump, the patient must input the precise number of grams of carbohydrates consumed. Some researchers are investigating the possibility of using image recognition analytics that will enable patients to take a picture of food on their plates and send the image to a neural network, which will analyze the picture and send the person a recommendation for the number of carbohydrates in the meal. Another factor that influences glucose levels, and thus insulin levels, is exercise. When the patient starts using a pump, he or she must figure out insulin sensitivity and record it in the pump. If the individual has a regular exercise routine, this information can also be programmed into the pump. The pump can remember patterns of eating, exercise, and insulin delivery for up to several weeks. Using all this data, algorithms calculate in real time the amount of insulin needed for both basal and bolus deliveries. Based on past patterns, new information, and probability calculations, the pump can predict low glucose readings and, when necessary, automatically suspend insulin delivery. If high glucose levels are predicted, the pump figures out how much additional insulin is needed and delivers it. For basal insulin, the adjustment can be automatic, but for an additional bolus, the patient must approve the amount of insulin. In all likelihood, bolus doses also will be automated in the future. Whether the pump is semiautonomous or autonomous, the patient effectively outsources analytics and decision making to the continuous glucose monitor and pump.

When I began to use the closed-loop system, my pump and I had to get to know each other. It had to learn my patterns of eating, sleeping, exercising, and glucose levels throughout the day and night, and I had to learn to trust the pump and let it do what it wants to do. More challenging, I had to learn to be willing to do what the pump wants when it wants me to do it. My pump really does have a mind of its own—it can be a harsh taskmaster that allows no disagreement.

All of this is very new. As I have noted, though crude forms of the insulin pump have been around since the

1960s, the first continuous glucose monitor was approved in 1999, and the monitor and the pump were only connected in 2016. These technological innovations have led to radical changes in the treatment of diabetes. A 2018 article reviewing recent research literature entitled "Artificial Intelligence for Diabetes Management and Decision Support" reports,

> Over the last decade, the entire paradigm of diabetes management has been transformed due to the integration of new technologies such as continuous glucose monitoring (CGM) devices and the development of the artificial pancreas (AP), along with the exploitation of data acquired by applying these novel tools. AI is attracting increased attention in this field because the amount of data acquired electronically from patients suffering from diabetes has grown exponentially. By means of complex and refined methods, AI has been shown to provide useful management tools to deal with these incremental repositories of data. Thus, AI has played a key role in the recognition of these systems as routine therapeutic aids for patients with diabetes.[21]

Once data from my pump have been uploaded to the cloud, my doctor as well as manufacturers and the helpline for the CGM and pump have access to it. My doctor analyzes the data and emails me instructions for any adjustments I need to make. This technology renders doctor visits and physical examinations virtually obsolete. If I have technical problems with the monitor or pump, trained educators are available 24/7 on the phone or online. This method of treatment has significant economic implications that have not yet been addressed. Unlike lawyers who charge in as little as five-minute increments and start the clock ticking as soon as they pick up the phone, so far doctors do not charge patients for analyzing their data, making recommendations, and contacting pharmacies for prescriptions. With a decline in the number of office visits, it is inevitable that these tele-services will soon be billed to patients.

Here, perhaps more than anywhere else, the question of who owns and who has access to data is very important. Responding to privacy concerns arising from the gradual adoption of electronic medical records, Congress passed the 1996 Health Insurance Portability and Accountability Act. This was intended to protect the privacy of medical records and to make it easier for people to change insurance companies by increasing the portability of their information. But an unintended consequence of the act has been to make it much harder for physicians and researchers to get access to the data they need. While I am sensitive to the problems associated with unauthorized access to any personal information, I am also acutely aware of the importance of Big Data for medical research and treatment. If a cure for diabetes and many other diseases is ever going to be found, it will require the willingness of the sick as well as the healthy to grant access to all their medical records.

Two other uses of the technologies I have been considering for the treatment of diabetes deserve consideration. My CGM and insulin pump are wearable devices, but they are not precisely the affective computers Picard and others are developing. There are times, however, when such devices would be enormously useful for diabetics. As we have seen, while long-term complications result from elevated glucose levels, low glucose levels can lead to the loss of consciousness, coma, and even death. When I am awake, I usually am able to feel when my glucose is low and take corrective measures, but some people cannot recognize dropping glucose levels, and this is very dangerous. There are clear physical signs of low glucose—rapid heartbeat and respiration, perspiration, pale complexion, loss of cognitive coherence, and, in my unusual case, visual hallucinations. Sometimes, for inexplicable reasons, the glucose level drops too fast for the pump's correction in insulin dosage to be effective quickly enough. When this happens, it is necessary to ingest or inject glucose immediately, but if the person is disoriented, he or she might not be able to do so. In these cases, a wearable computer could detect symptoms and notify the healthcare provider or send an alarm to the mobile phone of a parent, spouse, or friend who could intervene if the patient is incapacitated.

There is another possible solution to this and similar problems that has far-reaching implications for networking subjects. In the near future, I expect the closed loop between my CGM and pump, which are part of my personal area network, will be opened and connected directly to the all-encompassing Internet of Things and Internet of Bodies. This will enable the constant real-time transmission and reception of information that can be used for medical treatment and behavior modification. Wired bodies will be online 24/7/365; regardless of where they are, bodies will be able to communicate with other things and bodies in real time. Algorithms processing data on deep learning neural networks will detect problems before human beings can do so, calculate probabilities for alternative courses of action, and deliver recommendations to patients or, more likely, make decisions by themselves in real time. It is important to stress that these calculations will not depend solely on a person's individual data but will take into account information collected from the entire IoB as well as from the increasingly intelligent environment created by the rapid expansion of ubiquitous computing. When the algorithms are not adequate for the task, machines will autonomously produce more effective algorithms to monitor and treat patients.

It is necessary to recall the possibility of a new danger these developments will create—body hacking. Someone could hack into these networks to modify behavior or even to kill a person. For example, if I were connected to such networks, someone could kill me by cutting off or administering an overdose of insulin. I see no way of avoiding this danger—if Russians can already hack our elections, surely people intent on harm will be able to hack bodies. Nonetheless, I believe the risk of dying from the complications of diabetes far outweighs the risk of dying from body hacking. I'm staying plugged in.

The world is changing faster than our ability to comprehend it. Many of the developments I describe are already occurring even though most people remain unaware of them. While some of these ideas are speculative, they are well grounded in what is already actual or possible. I am no longer the self I had long believed myself to be. My body is not merely my own, but is connected to smart things and smart bodies without which I cannot exist. Like AlphaGo Zero making a completely original move, the algorithms programming the body know things no human being can know and do things physicians have never imagined doing. The networks on which these algorithms run are getting smarter faster and faster. As they become more intelligent, *I become relatively less intelligent until I become a prosthesis to what I had thought was my prosthesis.* As prostheses to prostheses and webs within webs become ever more interrelated, the Intranet of my Body, the Internet of Things, and the Internet of Bodies will intervolve in ways that can be neither predicted nor fully controlled. The question that remains is whether these developments pose a threat, an opportunity, or both.

5

Intervolutionary Future

often ask my students, "Do you think evolution stops with us and we are the last form of life on earth?" I tell them to think not only one hundred years into the future, but thousands, even millions of years ahead. Invariably, they say "No." When I ask, "Well, then, what comes next?," they fall silent. As Yogi once said, "It's tough to make predictions, especially about the future." One of the difficult truths that evolution teaches is that nothing lasts forever. Human being, like all other forms of life, is but a fleeting chapter in a much longer story whose beginning and end remain shrouded in mystery. People can no more imagine what will surpass them than dolphins and chimpanzees could have imagined *Homo sapiens*. Nevertheless, my "artificial" pancreas offers clues to what comes after the human.

Borrowing Heidegger's account of the craftsman who becomes aware of his tool and, correlatively, of himself when the tool breaks, I have argued that disease is the breakdown that reveals the body's structure and operation.

Through the analysis of the immune system and autoimmune disease, we have seen that the body is a network of networks that stores data and processes information. This Intranet is increasingly connected to the Internet of Things and the Internet of Bodies. The one who anticipated twenty-first-century relational networks that process information distributed throughout natural, social, and cultural systems is the nineteenth-century philosopher Hegel. His language is notoriously difficult, but his fundamental insight can be stated clearly and concisely: Hegel's system is a network of networks that mirrors the structure of the world and the place of human being in it. In this evolving web, everything is interrelated, and therefore to be is to be connected. While Hegel was fully conversant with the most advanced scientific work of his day being done in the fields of physics, chemistry, and biology, he could not have anticipated the extraordinary technological changes that have taken place in the nearly two centuries since he died. Nonetheless, his systematic vision offers the most useful perspective I know for understanding the new world now emerging. Writing during the early years of the Industrial Revolution, before the invention of the telegraph and telephone led to the wiring of the globe, Hegel did not adequately recognize the transformative effect of technology. It is, therefore, necessary to extend his insights to include the technological revolution currently unfolding.

Hegel's system consists of three integrally related parts: logic, nature, and spirit. If misunderstanding is to be avoided, it is essential to note that for Hegel, logic is not merely subjective or is not only inward mental activity; to the contrary, logic is the structural foundation of all natural,

144

social, and cultural processes. In *Science of Logic* (1812), he claims that metaphorically his logic is "the mind of God before the creation of the world." So understood, Hegel's logic translates the Christian doctrine of the Logos into a philosophical account of the rational ground of being. Reason is constitutive of subjects and objects as well as minds and bodies. Hegel has an idiosyncratic interpretation of logic, and his view of reason differs from the traditional accounts. In contrast to interpretations of reason based on the principle of noncontradiction, according to which something cannot be itself and its opposite at the same time, Hegel insists that everything is self-contradictory because opposites are interdependent and thus are mutually constitutive. This dialectical relation of opposites is what Hegel means by "spirit."

In his comprehensive *Encyclopedia of the Philosophical Sciences* (1817), Hegel makes the critical transition from nature (object) to spirit (subject) by analyzing disease. Simultaneously anticipating and reversing Heidegger's account of the tool, disease, Hegel argues, reveals the essence of life. Whereas for Heidegger the broken tool shows the separation between subject and object, for Hegel, disease reveals the necessary interrelation between subjects and things and subjects and other subjects. "The organism is in a *diseased* state when one of its systems or organs is *stimulated* into conflict with the inorganic potency of the organism. Through this conflict, the system or organ establishes itself in isolation, and by persisting in its particular activity in opposition to the activity of the whole, obstructs the fluidity of this activity, as well as the process by which it pervades all the moments of the whole." Disease, in other words, is a symptom of internal opposition in which one part of the organism is separated from the whole of which it should be an integral member. This "isolated determinateness is an individual [organ or system]," which attempts to assert its independent identity by excluding what initially appears to be other than itself (i.e., its other organs or systems)."[1] As we have discovered, while the immune system is based on the principle of noncontradiction—either self or other—autoimmune disease presupposes the principle of contradiction—both self and other. The abstract understanding of identity as opposed to and exclusive of otherness is misguided. Never simply itself by itself, every thing and every body is always already simultaneously itself and the other of itself. In the difficult language of *Science of Logic*,

> Identity is the reflection-into-self that is identity only as internal repulsion [*Abstossen*], and is the repulsion as reflection-into-self, repulsion, which immediately takes itself back into itself. Thus it is identity as difference that is identical with itself. But difference is only identical with itself in so far as it is not identity but absolute non-identity. But non-identity is absolute in so far as it contains nothing of its other but only itself, that is, in so far as it is absolute identity with itself. Identity, therefore, is *in its own self* absolute non-identity.[2]

This insight is the key to Hegel's entire system. Opposites are not externally related but are internally related in such a way that each becomes itself in and through the other and neither can be itself without the other. What appear to be sharply fixed boundaries are actually porous borders that lend identity—be it biological, psychological, or social—endless adaptability and fluidity. To heal disease, it is necessary to overcome oppositional identity and difference. "It is by means of the healing agent that the organism is excited into annulling the particular excitement in which the formal activity of the whole is fixed, and restoring the fluidity of the particular organ or system within the whole."[3] Healing restores life as the "universal fluid medium."[4]

In this sustaining matrix, everything is interdependent and intervolves: identity/difference, subject/object, mind/body, animate/inanimate, human/machine, natural/artificial, private/public, autonomy/heteronomy. Life is fractal, that is to say, it has the same structure at every level. Each individual is constituted and sustained in an extensive and intensive relational web that consists of a network of networks. Since subjects and objects are isomorphic, self-consciousness and nature mirror each other. In his *Phenomenology of Spirit* (1807), Hegel writes, "this is just how *self-consciousness* is constituted; it likewise distinguishes itself from itself without producing any distinction. Hence it finds in the observation of organic nature nothing else than a being of this kind. It finds itself as a thing, *as a life*, but makes a distinction between what it is itself and what it has found, a distinction, however, which is none."[5] Life is not something above or beyond individual living beings, but is nothing more than their vital interrelationship. Things that embody reason are *smart things*, and nature that reflects consciousness and self-consciousness is comprised of *smart bodies*, even if they do not know themselves as such.

Hegel rejects every form of dualism in which subjects are isolated from the world and act upon it externally; rather, human beings are integral parts of the natural order of things. Hegel describes this order as "objective spirit," which is the physical and material embodiment of the logic. In contemporary terms, objective spirit is distributed information that is coded, stored, and processed by computational machines ranging from molecules and cells to smart things and bodies. As Paul Ricoeur suggests, these codes, which can be genetic or cultural, "are 'programs' of behavior; like them, they confer form, order, and direction on life. But unlike genetic codes, cultural codes have been constructed in the collapsed zones of genetic regulation, and can prolong their efficiency only through a total reorganization of the coding system."[6] Since they share a common code, nature and society come to self-consciousness in and through human being's consciousness of them. Far from an external intervention, human action on the surrounding world is a self-reflexive process in which nature and society act upon themselves. By decoding and recoding the surrounding world, humans rewire themselves. All that is needed to complete this analysis is the inclusion of technology in this dialectical story.

To understand how Hegel's system illuminates the interrelation of the Intranet of the Body, the Internet of Things, and the Internet of Bodies, it is necessary to underscore five points. First, in living organisms order is internally emergent rather than externally imposed. Second, the relation between parts and whole is thoroughly *interactive*—the whole simultaneously emerges from the interplay of parts and acts back on these parts to constitute their differential identities. Third, the whole is an integrative *relational structure* that is the interplay of the parts. Fourth, while the

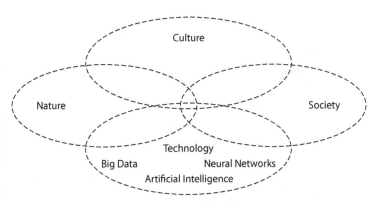

FIGURE 5.1 Nature—society—culture—technology.

whole provides a certain stability, it is not a fixed form but a *dynamic pattern* that changes constantly. And finally, this relational structure provides the *parameters of constraint* within which parts continue to develop. Since the whole is reconfigured as parts change, *whole and part are interdependent and intervolve.*

As I have suggested, Hegel's dialectical analysis subverts simple oppositions between natural and artificial, organism and mechanism, internal and external. It was Kant, not Hegel, who first understood that the constitutive principle of living organisms is *self-organization.* He makes this point by comparing biological organisms to mechanical watches. In a watch, "one part is certainly present for the sake of another, but it does not owe its presence to the agency of that other. For this reason, also, the producing cause of the watch and its form is not contained within the nature of this material, but lies outside the watch in a being that can act according to ideas of a whole which its causality makes possible." In organisms, by contrast, "every part is thought as *owing* its presence to the *agency* of all the remaining parts, and also as existing *for the sake of the others* and the whole, that is as an instrument, or organ. . . . Only under these conditions and upon these terms can such a product be an *organized* and *self-organized being*."[7]

In the years since Kant and Hegel were writing, the boundary separating organisms and machines has become porous. Organisms now appear to be information-processing machines and machines can create so-called artificial intelligence and even artificial life.[8] In fact, it is no longer clear what is artificial and what is not. Chilean biologists and neuroscientists Humberto Maturana and Franciso Varela coined the term *autopoiesis* to describe the processes of active *self-generation* and *self-maintenance*. Underscoring the importance of the principle of self-organization in biology, they argue that "living systems are machines that cannot be shown by pointing to their components. Rather, one must show their organization in a manner such that the way in which all their peculiar properties becomes obvious." Far from opposites, organisms and machines are symbiotic. More precisely, organisms are self-organizing systems that presuppose the effective operation of molecular information-processing machines. "*An autopoietic machine*," they write, "*is organized (defined as a unity) as a network of processes of production (transformation and destruction) of components that produces the components, which: (i) through their interactions and transformations continuously regenerate and realize the network of processes (relations) that produced them; and (ii) constitute it (the machine) as a concrete unity in the space in which they (the components) exist by specifying the topological domain of its relation as such a network."* Maturana and Varela offer what is, in effect, a gloss on Hegel's account of the interdependence of parts and whole when they argue that "an autopoietic machine continuously generates and specifies its own organization through its operation as a system of production of its own components, and does this in an endless turnover of components under conditions of continuous perturbations and compensation of perturbations."[9] This account of autopoiesis accurately describes the structure and operational logic among the Intranet of the Body, the Internet of Things, and the Internet of Bodies.

Autopoietic systems develop in emergent complex adaptive networks where negative and positive feedback loops join nature, society, culture, and technology in a ceaseless intervolutionary process. A change in any element in this network brings about changes in all the others. Since interiority and exteriority are cointerdependent, what appears to be a heteronomous relation with other things and bodies is actually an autonomous self-relation. As a result of this cointerdependence, technogenesis is anthropogenesis, and anthropogenesis is technogenesis. Once again, Stelarc's insight is suggestive; in an interview entitled "Extended-Body," he explains, "Technology has always been coupled with the evolutionary development of the body. Technology is what defines being human. It's not an antagonistic alien sort of object, it's part of our human nature. We shouldn't have a Frankensteinian fear of incorporating technology into the body, and we shouldn't consider our relationship to technology in a Faustian way—that we're somehow selling our soul because we're using these forbidden energies. My attitude is that technology is, and always has been, an appendage of the body."[10] And, I would add, the body is an appendage of technology. While Stelarc's performances effectively stage the activities of an extended body, he pays insufficient attention to the way neural networks, deep learning, and artificial intelligence create an extended mind. Furthermore, he does not acknowledge the likelihood that the interevolution of smart things and smart bodies will lead to new forms of life that surpass human being.

A consideration of how feedback loops connecting the Intranet of the Body, the Internet of Things, and the Internet of Bodies, which intersect in my "artificial" pancreas, are transforming human being can be clarified by examining the way in which technology has created extended minds and extended bodies. The activity of the mind can no more be limited to the operation of the brain within the skull than the activity of the body can be limited to the organism within the skin. In a world of ambient intelligence and ubiquitous computing, it is necessary to reconfigure the connections among mind, body, self, and world. In his book *Natural-Born Cyborgs: Minds, Technologies, and the Future of Human Intelligence*, Andy Clark, philosopher of logic and metaphysics, writes, "The notion of a real, central, yet wafer-thin self is a profound mistake. It is a mistake that blinds us to our real nature and leads us to radically undervalue and misconceive the roles of context, future, environment, and technology in the *constitution* of human persons. To face up to our true nature (soft selves, distributed decentralized coalitions) is to recognize the inextricable intimacy of self, mind, and world."[11]

The extended mind can be approached from two apparently opposite directions—moving from the inner to the outer, or moving from the outer to the inner. While everyone is familiar with warnings about videogames, iPhones, iPads, and other digital devices rewiring our brains, few people actually understand how this process works. Terrence Deacon presents one of the most instructive accounts of neuro- and cortical plasticity in his analysis of "the coevolution of language and the brain." Language, like writing, code, and algorithms, is a technology designed to store, process, and communicate information. Rather than regarding language as an epiphenomena of the brain's physiological structure, Deacon argues that the brain actually adapts to language. "The brain's wiring is determined by virtue of the interaction of information conveyed by its connections, so the way that information is analyzed ultimately becomes reflected in the way the brain regions are 'designed' by this activity." Brain and language are bound in a seemingly endless feedback loop—language wires and rewires the brain, which creates language. When understood in this way, Deacon's interpretation of language is similar to Saussure's *langue* and Hegel's Logos (i.e., logic). "I do not suggest that a disembodied thought acted to change the physical structure of our brains, as might a god in a mythical story, but I do suggest that the first use of symbolic reference by some distant ancestors changed how natural selection processes have affected hominid brain evolution ever since. So in a very real sense I mean that the physical changes that make us human are the incarnations, so to speak, of the process of using words."[12] Since language, codes, algorithms, and programs are not merely mental phenomena but are embodied in the world, the evolutionary process is inherently intelligible. Maurice Merleau-Ponty cites Hegel to underscore this point. "The mind of nature is a hidden mind. It is not produced in the form of mind itself; it is only mind for the mind which knows it: it is mind in itself, but not for itself."[13]

To appreciate the full impact of Deacon's argument, it is necessary to consider a broader range of technologies that transform human minds and bodies. Implants, transplants, and nanotechnology directly affect cognitive activity by altering physiological functions and changing neural connections. Smart devices, especially when networked, are dialectically related to both minds and bodies. Information processes distributed throughout the Intranet of the Body interact with distributed information processes in the Internet of Things and the Internet of Bodies. This expansive network of networks creates what Gregory Bateson labeled an "ecology of mind." "The individual mind is immanent but not only in the body. It is immanent also in pathways and messages outside the body; and there is a larger Mind of which the individual is only a subsystem. . . . What I am saying expands the mind outward . . . and these changes reduce the scope of the conscious self."[14]

The expanded mind not only extends from outer devices and processes to the inner recesses of what we once thought was our private self but also extends from apparent inwardness to outer networks without which it is impossible to think. Andy Clark and David Chalmers begin their hotly debated article "The Extended Mind" by asking, "Where does the mind stop and the rest of the world begin? The question invites two standard replies. Some accept the boundaries of skin and skull and say that what is outside the body is outside the mind. Others are impressed by arguments suggesting that the meaning of our words 'just ain't in the head,' and hold that its externalism about meaning carries over to an externalism about mind. We propose to pursue a third position. We advocate a very different sort of externalism: an active externalism, based on the active role of the environment in driving cognitive processes." Their argument turns on an important distinction between cognition and consciousness. While consciousness presupposes cognition, cognition does not necessarily presuppose consciousness. Many, if not most, cognitive processes are preconscious or even unconscious. Once cognition is distinguished from consciousness, it becomes possible to entertain the possibility of inanimate devices carrying out cognitive processes. Whether or not artificial intelligence ever achieves consciousness or self-consciousness, it is already undeniable that smart things and smart bodies are capable of cognition or quasi cognition. In developing their argument for the extended mind, Clark and Chalmers, like Deacon, take the technology of language as their point of departure. "The major burden of the coupling between agents is carried by language. Without language, we might be much more akin to discrete Cartesian 'inner' minds, in which high-level cognition relies largely on internal resources. But the advent of language has allowed us to spread this burden into the world. Language, thus construed, is not a mirror of our inner states but a complement to them. It serves as a tool whose role is to extend cognition in ways that on-board devices cannot." This expanded notion of the mind leads to a recasting of the boundaries of the self. "What, finally, of the self? Does the extended mind imply an extended self? It seems so. Most of us already accept that the self outstrips the boundaries of consciousness; my dispositional beliefs, for example, constitute in some deep sense part of who I am. If so, then these boundaries may also fall beyond the skin."[15]

From this point of view, people are "coupled" with computational devices in a way that creates a "cognitive loop" between the human mind and the environment. To illustrate this point, Clark and Chalmers take the example of an Alzheimer's patient named Otto who has a notebook that serves as an *aide de memoire*. In a more contemporary idiom, Otto has downloaded his memory into his notebook. This argument is at least as old as Plato's concern that writing would become a mental enhancement that would diminish humankind's memory capacity. The notebook is, of course, a metaphor for the proliferation of mind-expanding technologies that function as "epistemic artifacts" or "epistemic agents." Paul Smart upgrades Otto's notebook by expanding the analysis to digital "bio-external resources." Like Otto, Otto++ is "neurologically impaired."

> In order to ensure that he has access to relevant information, Otto++ installs an app that enables him to record important pieces of information. The app, however, does not store information locally on the device. Instead, it relies on a semantically enabled, cloud-based personal

data store that stores information in a linked data format. In order to access his personal data store, Otto++ installs an app that enables him to quickly retrieve important items of information using an intuitive graphical user interface. He also links his phone to his augmented reality glasses so that relevant information from his data store can be presented within his visual field.[16]

With the introduction of neural networks and deep learning, it becomes possible to customize and personalize Otto++'s memory in a way that makes it more reliable and therefore more useful. Within this expanding web, where, indeed, does the mind stop and the rest of the world begin?

In addition to the World Wide Web and the Internet of Things, social media extend the minds of individuals. Hutchins describes cognitive activity in social networks as "cognition in the wild." As we will see in our consideration of emerging complex adaptive networks, this interaction is not only between individuals and other individuals in his or her social network but also occurs at a meta-level independently of separate subjects. This meta-network emerges from networked selves and takes on a life of its own that transforms the individuals who created it. Hutchins argues,

> The proper unit of analysis for talking about cognitive change includes the socio-material environment of thinking. *Learning is adaptive reorganization in a complex system.* . . . This heavy interaction of internal and external structure suggests that the boundary between inside and outside, or between individual and context, should be softened. The apparent necessity of drawing such a boundary

is in part a side effect of the attempt to deal with the individual as an isolated unit of cognitive analysis without first locating the individual in a culturally constructed world. With the focus on a person who is actually engaged in culturally constructed world, let us soften the boundary of the individual and take the individual to be a very plastic kind of adaptive system.[17]

Soft boundaries create a two-way flow from outer to inner and inner to outer.

Since it is increasingly difficult to know where "natural" intelligence ends and "artificial" intelligence begins in environments of embedded sensors, with mobile devices that create environments of ubiquitous computing and distributed cognition, it is impossible to separate smart bodies and smart things. The interaction of the Intranet of the Body with the Internet of Things and the Internet of Bodies creates an extended body that is interdependent with the extended mind. Merleau-Ponty correctly maintains, "In recognizing that behavior has a meaning and depends upon the vital significance of situations, biological science is prohibited from conceiving of it as a thing in itself (*en soi*), which would exist, *partes extra partes, in* the nervous system or *on* the body; rather it sees *in* behavior an embodied dialectic that radiates over a milieu immanent to it."[18] When fully developed, the relation between body and milieu surpasses prosthetic relationships—as the opposition between the natural and the artificial is sublated, two become one. To understand how this hybrid is created, it is instructive to consider the apparently lowly example of termites and their nests.

Social insects like bees, wasps, and ants are well-known for cooperative activity through which they create extraordinary hives and nests that are extremely sophisticated and often more efficient than any human architect could design. In his book *The Extended Organism: The Physiology of Animal-Built Structures*, J. Scott Turner asks, are animal-built structures "best regarded as external to the animals that build them, or are they more properly considered parts of the animals themselves?" Answering his own question, he writes, "I am an advocate for the latter interpretation, but the argument I present in this book is one with a twist: that animal-built structures are properly considered organs of physiology, in principle no different from, and just as much a part of the organism as, the more conventionally defined organs such as kidneys, hearts, lungs, or livers."[19] Turner considers his analysis to be an extension of Richard Dawkins's argument about the extended phenotype. The function of the phenotype, Dawkins maintains, is not limited to synthesizing proteins but also includes the impact genes have on the environment. One of the examples he offers to illustrate his point is the way animals like beavers alter their environment by creating architectural structures like dams.[20] Elaborating Dawkins's suggestions, Turner argues that the symbiotic relation between termites and their nest is so close that they form a single organism.

The groundbreaking research that is the basis of Turner's analysis was published by Martin Lüscher in his 1961 article, "Air-conditioned Termite Nests." Lüscher points out that since most termites live in hostile environments, their survival depends on the ability to create dwellings that regulate the temperature and the moisture content of the air.

"Termites survive only because their elaborate social organization enables them to build nests in which they establish
the microclimate suited to their needs."[21] Termites are, in
effect, sophisticated "air-conditioning engineers." Nests,
which are built with a cardboardlike material made from
wood particles glued together with saliva and excrement,
can be as large as 16 feet in diameter and 16 feet tall, with
walls measuring between 16 and 23 inches. The nests have
multiple rooms including a cellar, an attic, rooms for culti-
vating and storing food, rooms for reproduction, and even
rooms for burying the dead. Termites' extreme sensitivity
to temperature and moisture fluctuations necessitated
the evolution of the ability to design and construct self-
regulating dwellings. Some species die within as little as
five hours if exposed to dry air. In order to avoid aridity,
nests draw moisture from the earth and cultivate fungus
whose fermentation process produces heat and releases
moisture. A medium-size colony consists of approximately
2 million termites that consume up to 240 liters of oxygen
(1,200 liters of air) a day. To provide a continuous flow of
clean air, the nests must include an elaborate circulation
system between the underground cellar and the attic at the
top of the nest.

Turner describes this intricate structure as a "colossal
heart-lung machine for the colony." This organismic
machine is self-regulating and inter-adaptive with the environment. According to Turner, "adaptation is not simply the
response of organisms to the environment: it also involves
the environment adapting to organism." Such inter-
adaptivity subverts the simple opposition between organism and milieu. What had appeared to be a fixed boundary

between inside and outside is actually an endless *process of exchange,* which resembles the formation and dissolution of whirlpools in a rushing river.

> It is precisely this "fuzzy" boundary between living and nonliving that is at the crux of the physiology of the extended phenotype. If the whirlpool can be nudged closer to the realm of the living by conferring upon it the ability to adaptively modify its environment, then what should we think about organisms that do the same? If an organism modifies its environment for adaptive purposes, is it fair to say that in so doing it confers a degree of livingness on its apparently inanimate surroundings? If we agree, just for the sake of argument, that it does, then the boundary between organism and NOT-organism, the boundary that seems so tangible—so obvious—to our senses of vision and touch, dissipates into an indistinct blur, much as a turbulent eddy merges imperceptibly into the water surrounding it.[22]

This interplay between organism and environment creates what Turner describes as a "superorganism."

E. O. Wilson and Bert Hölldobler develop the most extensive account of superorganisms in their studies of ant colonies. Drawing on Turner's discussion of termites, they explain, "Some social insects can build complex structures complete with air-conditioning and fortified 'castles.' But unlike human construction, there is no architect, no blueprint, no global design that governs the course of construction. Instead, nest structure *emerges* through the self-organization of multiple workers interacting with each other and with the environment they modify. . . . Social patterns and nest structures *emerge* from interactions between individuals guided by the same behavioral algorithms."[23] Worker termites and ants have no blueprint or plan to guide their actions. In a manner similar to the way the interactions of molecules and cells create a living organism, and dumb neurons in the brain create an agile mind, interactions among dumb termites and ants creates a vital organism that extends the body beyond the limits of every individual agent.

This understanding of social insects illuminates the world emerging in my insulin pump. The Intranet of my body is coupled to Internet of Things and the Internet of Bodies in a manner analogous to the relation among ants and between individual ants and the nest. Just as the nest functions as a heart-lung machine for individual termites, so the symbiotic relation among my body, my insulin pump, and broader networks of smart things and smart bodies extends "my" body beyond my skin. My body is no longer merely my own because it is interdependent with networks others create and sustain. I must continuously adapt to these networks as they are adapting to me. For me, as for termites, the boundary between organism and not-organism dissolves in networks of perpetual exchange.

These suggestive similarities notwithstanding, there would seem to be an obvious difference between termites and ants, on one hand, and, on the other, human beings. While insects are dumb and have no blueprints or plans, human beings appear to be smart and do seem to plan and self-consciously deliberate on their actions before making decisions. But human agents are not as smart as they think they are. While their actions may be purposeful, they do not really know what they are doing when they act. Actions of different individuals collide and ricochet back upon agents, often transforming what their deeds were intended to accomplish. With something like what Hegel describes as "the cunning of reason" and Adam Smith calls the "invisible hand" of the market, conflicting and complementary actions intersect to bring about results that were neither planned nor programmed. Like AlphaGo Zero's move 37, this aleatory event is a moment of unexpected creativity. Once again, the whole is greater than the sum of the parts. Through recursive negative and positive feedback loops, the whole adapts to the parts, which must adapt to the whole. In this way the interactions of networked intelligence and artificially intelligent agents give rise to superintelligence. *Superorganisms* and *superintelligence* are codependent emergent complex adaptive networks that form an intervolutionary process.

In a prescient series of lectures delivered at the Massachusetts Institute of Technology during the turbulent spring of 1968, economist and cognitive psychologist Herbert A. Simon explored what he described as "The Architecture of Complexity." His definition of complex systems is still quite useful. A complex system, he argues, is "one made up of a large number of parts that interact in a nonsimple way. In such systems, the whole is more than the sum of the parts, not in an ultimate, metaphysical sense, but in the important pragmatic sense that, given the properties of the parts and laws of their interaction, it is not a trivial matter to infer the properties of the whole."[24] In the years since Simon posed his argument, extensive research in a variety of fields has resulted in a considerably more sophisticated under-standing of complex systems. While the multiple branches of these investigations cannot be reduced to simple insights, common threads running through different analyses can be identified. In one of the most important developments, complexity theory has been used to interpret not only syn-chronic structures, but also diachronic development. David Depew and Bruce Weber argue that evolution itself evolves as an emergent complex adaptive process. They provide a definition of complex systems that is unusually concise yet very accurate. "Complex systems are systems that have a large number of components that can interact simultane-ously in a sufficiently rich number of parallel ways so that the system shows spontaneous self-organization and pro-duces global, emergent structures."[25] Given this definition, it is possible to identify the following characteristics of emergent complex adaptive systems:

1. Complex systems are comprised of many different parts, which are connected in multiple ways.
2. Diverse components can interact both serially and in par-allel to generate sequential as well as simultaneous effects and events.
3. Complex systems display spontaneous self-organization, which complicates interiority and exteriority in such a way that the line that is supposed to separate them becomes undecidable.
4. The structures resulting from self-organization emerge from but are not necessarily reducible to the interactivity of the components, elements, or agents in the system.

5. Though generated by local interactions, emergent properties tend to be global.

6. Inasmuch as self-organizing structures emerge spontaneously, complex systems are neither fixed nor static but develop or evolve. Such evolution presupposes that complex systems are both open and adaptive.

7. Emergence occurs in a narrow possibility space lying between conditions that are too ordered and too disordered. This boundary or margin is "the edge of chaos," which is always far from equilibrium.

Systems operating far from equilibrium are typically nonlinear. Microscopic and macroscopic operations and events are implicated in loops that involve both negative and positive feedback. Left to itself, negative feedback tends toward equilibrium by counterbalancing processes, which, if unchecked, can destroy the system. Positive feedback, by contrast, tends to disrupt equilibrium by increasing both the operational speed and heterogeneity of the components of the network. When positive feedback increases the speed of interaction among more and more diverse components, linear causality gives way to recursive relations in which effects are disproportionate to the causes from which they emerge. When this occurs, the system or network approaches the tipping point or, in more scientific terms, the condition of "self-organized criticality."

Physicist Per Bak has analyzed such events in great detail and has developed a theoretical explanation of them. "Complex behavior in nature," he argues, "reflects the tendency of large systems with many components to evolve into a poised 'critical' state, way out of balance, where minor disturbances may lead to events, called avalanches, of all sizes. Most of the changes take place through catastrophic events rather than by following a smooth gradual path. The evolution of this very delicate state occurs without design from any outside agent. The state is established solely because of the dynamical interactions among individual elements of the system: the critical state is *self-organized*."[26] When a system reaches the tipping point, the effect of individual events becomes unpredictable. While it is possible to know that at some point a significant change will occur, it is never possible to predict with certainty which event will tip the balance and upset the equilibrium. As the rate of change accelerates, ordered structures, systems, and networks tend to drift toward the edge of chaos, where an aleatory event can disturb, disrupt, and dislocate existing structures. Instead of a smooth continuous process, evolutionary development follows a pattern of what the late biologist Stephen Jay Gould described as "punctuated equilibrium." Periods of relative stability are interrupted by phase shifts that mark the *emergence* of new structures and reconfiguration of established networks. In this way, the event of emergence is the moment of creativity that is never possible apart from destruction.

Many informed and thoughtful scientists, engineers, and theorists are convinced that the technological developments I have been considering are rapidly bringing us to a tipping point. The most outspoken proponent of this point of view is Ray Kurzweil, who labels the quickly approaching tipping point "the Singularity." "The Singularity," he explains, "will represent the culmination of the merger of our biological thinking and existence with our technology, resulting in a world that is still human but transcends our biological roots. There will be no distinction, post-Singularity, between human and machine or between physical and virtual reality."[27] This development would mark a new phase in the process of evolution by bringing about the emergence of "superintelligence," which is structurally similar to superorganisms. Throughout history, biological change has occurred much more slowly than cultural change. The human brain, for example, has remained basically unchanged for centuries. However, as biological organisms become more machinic and machines become more biological, this will change. With the arrival of the technological singularity, Murray Shanahan argues, artificial intelligence will create superintelligence. "If the intellect becomes, not only the producer but also a product of technology, then a feedback cycle with unpredictable and potentially explosive consequences can result. For when the thing being engineered is intelligence itself, the very thing doing the engineering, it can set to work improving itself. Before long, according to the singularity hypothesis, the ordinary human is removed from the loop, overtaken by artificially intelligent machines or by cognitively enhanced biological intelligence and unable to keep pace."[28] While such speculations might seem fanciful, it is important to realize that high-speed self-programming computers already run algorithms that produce algorithms no human being could create. This is the way high-speed financial networks operate and how Amazon is able to deliver customized pop-up ads to consumers in real time. It is not inconceivable that these machines could develop a mind of their own that would be as incomprehensible to human beings as the mind of a bat.[29]

Larry Page and Sergey Brin have always insisted that Google is an artificial intelligence venture. Raffi Khatchadourian reports that "many of the world's largest tech companies are now locked in an AI arms race, purchasing other companies and opening specialized units to advance the technology. . . . After decades of pursuing narrow forms of AI, researchers are now seeking to integrate them into systems that resemble a general intellect. . . . One senior I.B.M. executive declared, 'The separation between human and machine is going to blur in a very fundamental way.'" The AI community is divided on the question of the feasibility of artificial intelligence becoming indistinguishable from human cognition. "Richard Sutton, a Canadian computer scientist . . . gives a range of outcomes: there is a ten-percent chance that A.I. will never be achieved, but a twenty-five-per-cent chance that it will arrive by 2030."[30]

While the prospect of AI that simulates human intelligence is daunting, the possibility of AI that surpasses human intelligence promises to be even more disorienting. The most prominent theorist of superintelligence is the philosopher Nick Bostrom, founding director of Oxford University's Future of Humanity Institute. Bostrom's approach to superintelligence is more inclusive than many AI researchers. He identifies three paths to superintelligence: "whole brain emulation, biological cognition, and human-machine interfaces, as well as networks and organizations."[31] The seemingly least disruptive path would be biological enhancement. Developments in biotechnology and the invention of increasingly sophisticated prostheses are already creating an interface in which the human and the machine can no longer be clearly distinguished. As the contributors to the illuminating volume *Medical Enhancement and Posthumanity* make clear, advances in transplant technology, genetic engineering, neuroscience, and nanotechnology are changing organisms in ways that push the human to the edge of the posthuman.[32] In the most radical example of medical enhancement to date, Dr. Ren Xiaoping, an orthopedic surgeon in Harbin, China, is attempting "full-body transplants." This procedure might better be described as a "brain transplant," which presupposes the separation of mind and brain/body that informs so much posthuman theory and discourse. Dr. Ren was trained at the universities of Louisville and Cincinnati and assisted at the first hand transplant performed in the United States in 1999. In a 2016 *New York Times* article, Didi Kirsten Tatlow explains that Ren's plan is "to remove two heads from two bodies, connect the blood vessels of the body of the deceased donor and the recipient head, insert a metal plate to stabilize the new neck, bathe the spinal cord nerve endings in a gluelike substance to aid regrowth and finally sew up the skin." According to Tatlow, Ren is not the only one experimenting with this procedure. "Dr. Sergio Canavero of the Turin Advance Neuromodulation Group in Italy, is a prominent advocate, and scientists at the Institute of Theoretical and Experimental Biophysics at the Russian Academy of Sciences are also researching aspects of the procedure."[33]

Less dramatic but no less significant is what Bostrom describes as "whole brain emulation," also known as "uploading." This approach involves a combination of neuroscience with hardware and software engineering. Bostrom

169

identifies three prerequisites for whole brain emulation. "*Scanning*: high-throughput microscopy with sufficient resolution and detection of relevant properties; (2) *translation*: automated image analysis to turn raw scanning data into an interpreted three-dimensional model of relevant neurocomputational elements; and (3) *simulation*: hardware powerful enough to implement the resultant computational structure." Bostrom thinks that the theoretical and practical requirements are in place for successful brain emulation in the near future.

The most intriguing possibility Bostrom presents involves ever-expanding global networks, which create the conditions for superintelligence as an emergent phenomenon that becomes virtually inevitable with growing connectivity and complexity.

> A more plausible version of the scenario would be that the Internet accumulates improvements through the work of many people over many years—work to engineer better search and information filtering algorithms, more powerful data representation formats, more capable autonomous software agents, and more efficient protocols governing the interactions between such bots— and that myriad incremental improvements eventually create the basis for some more unified form of web intelligence. It seems at least conceivable that such a web-based cognitive system, supersaturated with computer power and all other resources needed for explosive growth save for one crucial ingredient, could, when the final missing constituent is dropped into the cauldron, blaze up with superintelligence.[34]

In this version, superintelligence is structurally identical to superorganisms.

Before proceeding to a critical assessment of superintelligence, it is important to underscore an assumption underlying these speculations. Ever since the earliest days of information theory, it has been common to value pattern over stuff. Katherine Hayles identifies this presupposition as the foundation of theoretical posthumanism. "The posthuman view privileges information pattern over material instantiation, so that embodiment in a biological substrate is seen as an accident of history rather than an inevitability of life."[35] This claim leads to two problematic conclusions. First, if information and, by extension, intelligence could be separated from matter and biological bodies, the ancient dream of immortality might become technologically feasible. Second, if mind can be uploaded, software engineers will become latter-day Gnostics, who crack the code that enables them to drop their bodies, leave Earth, and rise through the celestial spheres. This is precisely Kurzweil's dream.

> Once a planet yields a technology-creating species and that species creates computation (as has happened here), it is only a matter of a few centuries before its intelligence saturates the matter and energy in its vicinity, and it begins to expand outward at at least the speed of light (with some suggestions of circumventing this limit). Such a civilization will then overcome gravity (through exquisite and vast technology) and other cosmological forces—or, to be fully accurate, it will maneuver and control these forces—and engineer the universe it wants. This is the goal of the Singularity.[36]

171

Remember, Kurzweil is not some crazed crackpot; rather, he is the director of engineering at Google, holds twenty-one honorary doctorates, has received awards from three United States presidents, was named by PBS as "one of sixteen revolutionaries who made America," and has been described by *Forbes* as "the rightful heir to Thomas Edison."

Brin and Page as well as other Silicon Valley scientists, engineers, and entrepreneurs share Kurzweil's vision. Some are even preparing for superintelligence's arrival by developing a strategy for leaving Earth. The goal of Jeff Bezos's and Elon Musk's space programs is not primarily to make money from space tourism but to develop the means to colonize the universe with conscious and self-conscious artificial intelligence when Earth becomes uninhabitable. "Unhampered by earthly biological needs," Shanahan explains, "and psychologically untroubled by the prospect of thousands of years of traveling through interstellar space, self-reproducing superintelligent machines would be in a good position to colonize the galaxy. From a large enough perspective, it might be seen as human destiny to facilitate this future, even though (unenhanced) humans themselves are physically and intellectually too feeble to participate in it."[37]

Even the most starry-eyed visionaries acknowledge the potential danger of runaway superintelligence. Bostrom goes so far as to suggest that superintelligence could pose what he describes as an "existential threat" to the human race. He is not alone in his fear of the possible outcome of accelerating and proliferating AI. Leading figures ranging from Stephen Hawking and Bill Gates to Elon Musk and Bill Joy have raised the prospect of a Frankenstein scenario in which intelligent machines take over the human world and render human beings first extraneous and eventually extinct. For such critics, superintelligence presents a danger as great as nuclear weapons. In a widely influential 2000 *Wired* magazine article entitled "Why the Future Doesn't Need Us," Joy, co-founder of Sun Microsystems, sounded the alarm. "We have the possibility not just of weapons of mass destruction but of knowledge-enabled mass destruction (KMD), this destruction is amplified by the power of self-replication." "Uncontrolled self-replication in these technologies," he claims, "runs a much greater risk: a risk of substantial damage in the physical world."[38] Bostrom is fully aware of this danger and argues that the "treacherous turn" will occur when AI begins to behave cooperatively. Running on machines whose complexity exceeds the complexity of the human brain at speeds far beyond the capacity of human beings, collective superintelligence might develop consciousness and even self-consciousness, which would enable it to evolve in unpredictable and uncontrollable ways. "Without knowing anything about the detailed means that a super-intelligence would adopt," Bostrom reflects, "we can conclude that a superintelligence—at least in the absence of intellectual peers and in the absence of effective safety measures arranged by humans in advance—would likely produce an outcome that would involve reconfiguring terrestrial resources into whatever structures might maximize the realization of its goals. Any concrete scenario we develop can at best establish a lower bound on how quickly and efficiently the superintelligence could achieve such an outcome. It remains possible that the superintelligence would find a shorter path to its preferred destination."[39] In this postbiological world, human beings face short-term slavery to the machines they have created and long-term extinction.

Such a scenario is not inevitable—the artificial pancreas I wear on my belt teaches different lessons about the world emerging in our midst. Kurzweil's analysis of the Singularity represents the latest version of the traditional view of technology as an expression of *man's* will to power or will to mastery. After mastering death by escaping the body, the next challenge becomes colonizing the universe. Kurzweil predicts, "Ultimately, the entire universe will become saturated with our intelligence. This is the destiny of the universe. We will determine our fate rather than have it determined by current 'dumb,' simple, machinelike forces that rule celestial mechanics."[40] When the universe is saturated with *our* intelligence, Heidegger's prediction becomes true: "everywhere *man* turns he sees only himself."[41] Down this path surely lies destruction.

Without in any way denying possible dangers in these new technologies, it is important to realize that they harbor creative as well as destructive possibilities. French philosopher and physician Georges Canguilhem points to another path when he writes, "The answer I am tempted to offer would insist on showing that technology allows man to live in continuity with life, as opposed to a solution that would see human kind as living in a state of rupture for which we ourselves are responsible because of science."[42]

Diabetes has taught me that I am never only myself, but am always also other than myself. As my pump and I have gotten to know each other, and we have learned to live together, I have discovered that my body extends beyond itself. The Intranet of my body, the Internet of Things, and the Internet of Bodies share a common language and therefore are able to communicate with each other. Sometimes we misunderstand each other and must recalibrate. My pump is always calculating, thinking, and talking to my body as well as to other smart things even if I am not. When I misread a glucose level or miscalculate my bolus dosage, my pump catches my mistake and corrects the error. Sometimes my pump asks for my advice, most of the time it does not. The network of networks that envelops me forms an emerging complex adaptive network in which something like a superorganism and superintelligence are already developing. I have become a node in this meta-network and no longer can live without it. Just as mind and body cannot be separated, so superorganism and superintelligence are interdependent and intervolve. I do not impose my intelligence on a recalcitrant world or resistant others; to the contrary, I am but a fleeting moment in a process that both includes and surpasses me. Body and mind I once thought were my own, I now realize are expressions of an intelligence that is neither simply natural nor merely artificial. As sentient environments and distributed cognition continue to expand, I along with all other smart things and smart bodies contribute to the complex intervolutionary process that continuously shapes everything and everyone.

To the question I ask my students—Do you think evolution stops with us and we are the last form of life?—my answer is a resounding "No!" Human being, like every other form of life, is but a single chapter in a much longer story whose beginning and end forever elude our grasp.

Though we cannot know with certainty what comes next, I suspect that in the years to come human beings and machines will become even more closely interrelated until the so-called natural and so-called artificial become indistinguishable. AI will become part of "my" mind, and what had been prostheses will become organs of "my" body. Then I will no longer have to wear "my" pancreas on my belt. At this tipping point, the form of life that once was known as human will intervolve into something we cannot imagine. "My" pump and the networks it supports and that support it have allowed me to participate in a process Hegel aptly describes as "the arising and passing away that does not arise and pass away" longer than I would have been able to without them.[43] This is not immortality, but it is enough for me as I give way to whatever comes next.

Notes

1. Our Bodies Our Selves

1. Samuel Beckett, *The Unnamable* (New York: Grove, 1958), 179.
2. Martin Heidegger, "The Provenance of Art and the Destination of Thought," *Journal of British Society for Phenomenology* 44, no. 2: 125, 123.
3. Martin Heidegger, *Being and Time*, trans. John Macquarrie and Edward Robinson (New York: Harper and Row, 1962), 422.
4. In the next chapter I will explain this process in more detail.
5. Michael Bliss, *The Discovery of Insulin* (Chicago: University of Chicago Press, 2007), 20. This book is the basis of an informative documentary film, *Glory Enough for All*.
6. Thomas Burton, "FDA Says Medtronic Insulin Pumps Pose Cybersecurity Risk," *Wall Street Journal*, June 27, 2018.
7. Shoshana Zuboff, *The Age of Surveillance Capitalism: The Fight for a Human Future at the New Frontier of Power* (New York: Public Affairs, 2019), 30.
8. Zuboff, 242–43.
9. Quoted in Zuboff, 98.
10. I will consider some of these initiatives in chapter 3.
11. *IDF Diabetes Atlas* (Brussels: International Diabetes Federation, 2017), 6. The information and statistics in the following pages are drawn from this report.

12. I will consider the reasons for this development in the next chapter.

13. Ken Alltucker, "Struggling to Stay Alive: Rising Insulin Prices Cause Diabetics to Go to Extremes," *USA Today*, March 27, 2019.

14. Jan Klein, *Immunology: The Science of Self-Nonself Discrimination* (New York: Wiley, 1982).

2. Intranet of the Body

1. Søren Kierkegaard, *The Sickness Unto Death,* trans. Howard and Edna Hong (Princeton: Princeton University Press, 1980), 23.

2. Susan Sontag, *Illness as Metaphor* (New York: Doubleday, 1989), 3.

3. Sontag, 4.

4. Ferdinand de Saussure, "Course in General Linguistics," in *Deconstruction in Context*, ed. Mark C. Taylor (Chicago: University of Chicago Press, 1986), 156.

5. Epitopes play a critical role in the immune system. They are the part of antigen molecules to which an antibody attaches itself. I will explain how the antibody-antigen relationship works later in this chapter.

6. Giorgio Prodi, "Signs and Codes in Immunology," in *The Semiotics of Cellular Communication in the Immune System*, ed. Eli Sercarz, F. Celaea, N. Mitchison, and T. Tada (New York: Springer, 1988), 57–58, 56.

7. Anthony Wilden, *System and Structure: Essays in Communication and Exchange* (London: Tavistock, 1972), 202–3.

8. Donna Haraway, *Simians, Cyborgs, and Women: The Reinvention of Nature* (New York: Routledge, 1991), 228.

9. I will consider the final metaphor for the immune system and autoimmunity—the Internet—after I have considered the biochemistry of the immune system.

10. Warwick Anderson and Ian Mackay, *Intolerant Bodies: A Short History of Autoimmunity* (Baltimore: Johns Hopkins University Press, 2014), 79–80.

11. Emily Martin, *Flexible Bodies: Tracking Immunity in American Culture from the Days of Polio to the Age of AIDS* (Boston: Beacon, 1994), 53, 50.

12. Peter Sloterdijk, *Spheres: Bubbles, Microspherology*, trans. Wieland Hoban (New York: Semiotext[e], 2011), 68–69.

13. Niels K. Jerne, "The Natural Selection Theory of Antibody Forma-
    tion," in *Phage and the Origins of Molecular Biology* (Cold Spring Har-
    bor, NY: Cold Spring Harbor Laboratory of Quantitative Biology,
    1966), 301.

14. Haraway, *Simians, Cyborgs, and Women*, 222–23.

15. Irun Cohen, "The Self, the World, and Autoimmunity," *Scientific
    American*, April 1988, 55.

16. Jacques Derrida, *Specters of Marx: The State of the Debt, the Work of
    Mourning, and the New International*, trans. Peggy Kamuf (New York:
    Routledge, 1994), 141.

17. N. K. Jerne, "Towards a Network Theory of the Immune System,"
    Annals of Allergy, Asthma, and Immunology (Paris), January 1974, 125
    C(1–2), 382.

18. Jerne, 387.

19. I will consider complex networks in more detail in chapter 5. For an
    examination of these developments, see my book, *The Moment of
    Complexity: Emerging Network Culture* (Chicago: University of Chicago
    Press, 2001).

20. Francisco Varela, Antonio Coutinho, Bruno Dupire, and Nelson Vaz,
    "Cognitive Networks Immune, Neural, and Otherwise," in *Theoretical
    Immunology*, ed. Alan S. Peterson (New York: Addison-Wesley, 1988),
    360–61.

179

3. Internet of Things

1. Eric Topol, *Deep Medicine: How Artificial Intelligence Can Make Healthcare Human Again* (New York: Basic Books, 2019), 74. For Kasparov's
   own account, written years later, see *Deep Thinking: Where Machine
   Intelligence Ends and Human Creativity Begins* (London: John Murray,
   2017).

2. Alan Turing, "Intelligent Machinery, a Heretical Theory," https://
   fermatslibrary.com/s/intelligent-machinery-a-heretical-theory.

3. Alan Turing, "Computing Machinery and Intelligence," https://www
   .csee.umbc.edu/courses/471/papers/turing.pdf. The word *computer*
   originally referred to people who carried out routine calculations. In

spite of Turing's use of the masculine pronoun in this passage, in the years before electronic computers this was considered to be clerical work and most of the computers were women.

4. Katherine Hayles, "Traumas of Code," *Critical Inquiry* 1, no. 33 (Autumn 2006): 136–57.

5. Joshua Cohen, *Book of Numbers* (New York: Random House, 2015), 98.

6. Georges Canguilhem, *A Vital Rationalist: Selected Writings*, ed. Francois Delaporte (New York: Zone, 1994), 316.

7. Turing, "Computing Machinery and Intelligence."

8. Yuval Noah Harari, *Homo Deus* (New York: Harper Collins, 2016), 348.

9. Edgar Allan Poe, "Maelzel's Chess Player, https://www.eapoe.org/works/essays/maelzel.htm, 1.

10. I will discuss Babbage's Difference Machine and Analytic Machine further on in this chapter.

11. Poe, "Maelzel's Chess Player," 2.

12. Alan Turing, "Digital Computers Applied to Games," http://eolo.cps.unizar.es/docencia/doctorado/Articulos/ArticulosFamosos/1953%20Alan%20Turing-Digital%20Computers%20Applied%20to%20Games%20in%20book%20Bowden-FasterThanThought.pdf, 289.

13. Edwin Hutchins, *Cognition in the Wild* (Cambridge, MA: MIT Press, 2000), 365.

14. Turing, "Computing Machinery and Intelligence."

15. See, for example, Daniel Halacy, *Charles Babbage: Father of the Computer* (New York: Cromwell-Collier, 1970).

16. Quoted in Douglas Hofstadter, *Gödel, Escher, Bach: An Eternal Golden Braid* (New York: Vintage, 1980), 25.

17. Turing, "Computing Machinery and Intelligence."

18. Turing.

19. Topol, *Deep Medicine*, 79.

20. Terrence Deacon, *The Symbolic Species: The Co-evolution of Language and the Brain* (New York: Norton, 1997), 131.

21. Nicholas Thompson, "An AI Pioneer Explains the Evolution of Neural Networks," https://www.wired.com/story/ai-pioneer-explains-evolution-neural-networks/, 3–4.

22. https://deepmind.com/about/.

23. Volodymyr Mnih et al., "Human-Level Control Through Deep Rein-forcement Learning," *Nature* 518 (February 2015): 529.

24. David Silver et al., "Mastering the Game of Go Without Human Knowl-edge," *Nature* 550 (October 2017): 358.

25. This citation is from the film *AlphaGo Zero*, https://www.alphagomovie.com/.

26. Silver et al., "Mastering the Game of Go Without Human Knowl-edge," 358.

27. Kai-Fu Lee, *AI Superpowers: China, Silicon Valley, and the New World Order* (New York: Houghton Mifflin Harcourt, 2018), 3.

28. https://deepmind.com/about/.

29. "Personal Data: The Emergence of a New Asset Class," an initiative of the World Economic Forum in collaboration with Bain & Co., Janu-ary 2001, 5.

30. Shoshana Zuboff, *The Age of Surveillance Capitalism: The Fight for a Human Future at the New Frontier of Power* (New York: Public Affairs, 2019), 64, 77.

31. Samuel Greengard, *The Internet of Things* (Cambridge, MA: MIT Press, 2015), 122.

32. Greengard, 13.

33. Quoted in Greengard, 59.

34. Lee, *AI Superpowers*, 19.

35. Mark Weiser, "The Computer for the Twenty-first Century," *Scientific American*, September 1991, 94, 100.

36. Zuboff, *The Age of Surveillance Capitalism*, 5. For a description of the Aware Home project, see the website: https://gvu.gatech.edu/research/labs/aware-home-research-initiative.

37. Zuboff, *Surveillance Capitalism*, 239, 293.

38. As my comments have suggested, Zuboff's *The Age of Surveillance Cap-italism* is a major contribution to our understanding of changes now occurring. She is, however, consistently critical and makes little or no effort to consider how these technologies can be used in more benefi-cial ways.

39. Joseph Paradiso, "Our Extended Sensoria: How Humans Will Connect with the Internet of Things," https://www.bbvaopenmind.com/en

181

/articles/our-extended-sensoria-how-humans-will-connect-with-the
-internet-of-things/.

4. Internet of Bodies

1. David Wills, *Prosthesis* (Stanford: Stanford University Press, 1995), 12–13.

2. Geeta Dayal, "For Extreme Artist Stelarc, Body Mods Hint at Humans' Possible Future," https://www.wired.com/2012/05/stelarc-performance -art/.

3. Stelarc, "Ping Body: An Internet Actuated and Uploaded Performance," http://www.medienkunstnetz.de/works/ping-body/. For a helpful collection on Stelarc's work, see Marquard Smith, ed., *Stelarc: The Monograph* (Cambridge, MA: MIT Press, 2005).

4. Ernesto Rodriguez Leal, "Robotics and the Internet of Bodies," https:// medium.com/pandemonio/robotics-and-the-internet-of-bodies -fdd073631ebb.

5. https://www.cbinsights.com/research/report/google-strategy -healthcare/.

6. https://www.cbinsights.com/research/report/google-strategy -healthcare/.

7. Sandip Panesar, "The Surgical Singularity Is Approaching," https:// blogs.scientificamerican.com/observations/the-surgical-singularity-is -approaching/.

8. Personal conversation. Daisuke Wakabayashi, "Google and the University of Chicago Are Sued Over Data Sharing," *New York Times*, June 26, 2019. I will return to this issue later in this chapter.

9. Eric Topol, *Deep Medicine: How Artificial Intelligence Can Make Healthcare Human Again* (New York: Basic Books, 2019), 115–16.

10. "The Future of Medicine," Jacobs Institute, University of Buffalo, November 1, 2017, https://bnmc.org/future-medicine-book-inspired -jacobs-institute/.

11. I will consider these applications in relation to diabetes care in what follows.

12. "The Future of Medicine."

13. Topol, *Deep Medicine*, 166.

14. Antonio Damasio, *The Feeling of What Happens: Body and Emotion in the Making of Consciousness* (New York: Harcourt Brace, 1999), 172.

15. Rosalind Picard, *Affective Computing* (Cambridge, MA: MIT Press, 1997), xiii.

16. Picard, 47. At the same time Picard was developing affective computing devices, her MIT colleagues Cynthia Breazeal and Rodney Brooks were working on humanoid robots that were emotionally responsive.

17. For a description of these projects as well as other work going on in the laboratory, see https://affect.media.mit.edu/projects.php.

18. Picard, *Affective Computing*, 16.

19. http://rogersgroup.northwestern.edu/.

20. Stelarc, "Ping Body."

21. Gunther Eysenbach, ed., "Artificial Intelligence for Diabetes Management and Decision Support: Literature Review," *Journal of Internet Research* 20, no. 5 (May 2018): e10775.

5. Intervolutionary Future

1. G. W. F. Hegel, *Philosophy of Nature*, trans. Michael Petry (New York: Humanities, 1970), 3:193, 199.

2. G. W. F. Hegel, *Science of Logic*, trans. A. V. Miller (New York: Humanities, 1969), 413.

3. Hegel, *Philosophy of Nature*, 3:202.

4. G. W. F. Hegel, *Phenomenology of Spirit*, trans. A. V. Miller (New York: Oxford University Press, 1977), 107.

5. Hegel, *Phenomenology*, 157.

6. Quoted in Bernard Stiegler, *Technics and Time, 1: The Fault of Epimethes*, trans. Richard Beardsworth and George Collins (Stanford: Stanford University Press, 1998), 138.

7. Immanuel Kant, *Critique of Judgment*, trans. James Meredith (New York: Oxford University Press, 1973), 21–22.

8. For discussions of artificial life, see Christopher Langton, ed., *Artificial Life*, Santa Fe Institute Studies (Reading, MA: Addison-Wesley, 1989, 1994), vols. 6, 17, and Steven Levy, *Artificial Life: A Report from the Frontier Where Computers Meet Biology* (New York: Random House, 1993).

9. Humberto Maturana and Francisco Varela, *Autopoiesis and Cognition: The Realization of the Living* (Boston: Reidel, 1980), 78–79.

10. Stelarc, "Extended-Body: Interview with Stelarc," https://web.stanford .edu/dept/HPS/stelarc/a29-extended_body.html.

11. Andy Clark, *Natural-Born Cyborgs: Minds, Technologies, and the Future of Human Intelligence* (New York: Oxford University Press, 2003), 139.

12. Terrence Deacon, *The Symbolic Species: The Co-evolution of Language and the Brain* (New York: Norton, 1997), 221, 322.

13. Maurice Merleau-Ponty, *The Structure of Behavior*, trans. Alden Fisher (Boston: Beacon, 1963), 161.

14. Gregory Bateson, *Steps to an Ecology of Mind* (New York: Chandler, 1972),

15. Andy Clark and David Chalmers, "The Extended Mind," *Analysis* 58, no. 1 (1998): 7, 18.

16. Paul Smart, "Emerging Digital Technologies: Implications for Extended Conceptions of Cognition and Knowledge," in J. Adam Carter, Andy Clark, and Jasper Kallerstrup, eds., *Extended Epistemology* (New York: Oxford University Press, 2018), 279. See also Richard Menary, ed., *The Extended Mind* (Cambridge, MA: MIT Press, 2010).

17. Edwin Hutchins, *Cognition in the Wild* (Cambridge, MA: MIT Press, 2000), 289, 288.

18. Merleau-Ponty, *The Structure of Behavior*, 161.

19. J. Scott Turner, *The Extended Organism: The Physiology of Animal-Built Structures* (Cambridge, MA: Harvard University Press, 2000), 1–2.

20. See Richard Dawkins, *The Extended Phenotype* (New York: Oxford University Press, 1999).

21. Martin Lüscher, "Air-Conditioned Termite Nests," *Scientific American* 205, no. 1 (July 1961): 138. I have drawn details about termites and their nests from this article.

22. Turner, *The Extended Organism*, 195, 211, 6.

23.   Bert Hölldobler and E. O. Wilson, *The Superorganism: The Beauty, Elegance, and Strangeness of Insect Societies* (New York: Norton, 2009), 473.

24.   Herbert A. Simon, "The Architecture of Complexity," in *The Sciences of the Artificial* (Cambridge, MA: MIT Press, 1969), 86.

25.   David Depew and Bruce Weber, *Darwinism Evolving: Systems Dynamics of the Genealogy of Natural Selection* (Cambridge, MA: MIT Press, 1995), 437.

26.   Per Bak, *How Nature Works: The Science of Self-Organized Criticality* (New York: Springer, 1969), 1–2.

27.   Ray Kurzweil, *The Singularity Is Near: When Humans Transcend Biology* (New York: Viking, 2005), 9.

28.   Murray Shanahan, *The Technological Singularity* (Cambridge, MA: MIT Press, 2015), xvi.

29.   See Thomas Nagel, "What Is It Like to Be a Bat?," *Philosophical Review* 83, no. 4 (October 1974): 435–50.

30.   http://www.newyorker.com/magazine/2015/11/23/doomsday -invention-artificial-intelligence-nick-bostrom.

31.   Nick Bostrom, *Superintelligence: Paths, Dangers, Strategies* (New York: Oxford University Press, 2014), 22.

32.   Bert Gordijn and Ruth F. Chadwick, *Medical Enhancement and Posthumanity* (New York: Springer, 2008).

33.   Didi Kirsten Tatlow, "Doctor's Plan for Full-Body Transplants Raises Doubts Even in China," *New York Times*, June 11, 2016.

34.   Bostrom, *Superintelligence*, 49.

35.   Katherine Hayles, *How We Became Posthuman: Virtual Bodies in Cybernetics, Literature, and Informatics* (Chicago: University of Chicago Press, 1999), 2.

36.   Kurzweil, *The Singularity Is Near*, 364.

37.   Shanahan, *The Technological Singularity*, 157.

38.   Bill Joy, "Why the Future Doesn't Need Us," *Wired*, April 2000.

39.   Bostrom, *Superintelligence*, 99.

40.   Kurzweil, *The Singularity Is Near*, 29.

41.   This interpretation of the will to power and the assumption that intelligence and mind can be separated from their so-called biological substrate is highly gendered. See, for example, Kate Crawford,

"Artificial Intelligence's White Guy Problem," *New York Times*, June 25, 2016.

42. Georges Canguilhem, "Machine and Organism," https://monoskop.org/images/7/7d/Canguilhem_Georges_1952_1992_Machine_and_Organism.pdf.

43. Hegel, *Phenomenology of Spirit*, 27.

Index

Seeing Silence

Abiding Grace: Time, Modernity, Death

Last Works: Lessons in Leaving

Speed Limits: Where Time Went and Why We Have So Little Left

Recovering Place: Reflections on Stone Hill

*Rewiring the Real: In Conversation with William Gaddis, Richard Powers,
    Mark Danielewski, and Don DeLillo*

Refiguring the Spiritual: Beuys, Barney, Turrell, Goldsworthy

Crisis on Campus: A Bold Plan for Reforming Our Colleges and Universities

Field Notes From Elsewhere: Reflections on Dying and Living

After God

Mystic Bones

Confidence Games: Money and Markets in a World Without Redemption

Grave Matters, with Dietrich Christian Lammerts

The Moment of Complexity: Emerging Network Culture

About Religion: Economies of Faith in Virtual Culture

The Picture in Question: Mark Tansey and the Ends of Representation

Critical Terms for Religious Studies

Hiding

Imagologies: Media Philosophy, with Esa Saarinen

The Real: Las Vegas, Nevada, with Jose Marquez

Nots

Disfiguring: Art, Architecture, Religion

Michael Heizer: Double Negative

Tears

Altarity

Deconstruction in Context: Literature and Philosophy

Erring: A Postmodern A/Theology

Deconstructing Theology

Journeys to Selfhood: Hegel and Kierkegaard

Unfinished . . . : Essays in Honor of Ray L. Hart

Religion and the Human Image, with Carl Raschke and James Kirk

Kierkegaard's Pseudonymous Authorship: A Study of Time and the Self